Artificial

Intelligence (AI)

vs

The Medical Staff

The Future of Healthcare

MANU SEKODI

Table of contents

Introduction

Background to the growing integration of artificial intelligence in the healthcare sector.

Over the last few decades, technological advances have significantly transformed the way we approach healthcare. Among these advances, artificial intelligence (AI) is emerging as one of the most revolutionary and promising technologies in the medical field. The increasing integration of AI into healthcare is the result of a combination of factors that have shaped the context for this transformation:

1. **Medical data explosion:** With the increasing digitisation of health records and the widespread use of connected medical devices, a massive amount of medical data has been generated and stored. The manual analysis and interpretation of this data is often beyond the capabilities of healthcare professionals, which is where AI can come in to help extract useful information and make more informed decisions.

2. **Increased computing power:** Advances in computing and algorithms have enabled AI systems to rapidly process huge volumes of data. This now makes it possible to apply machine learning and deep learning models to solve complex problems in medicine.

3. **Improved algorithm performance:** Researchers have made significant advances in the development of machine learning and deep learning algorithms, enabling AI to become more accurate and efficient in its predictions and diagnoses.

4. The needs of an ageing population : In many parts of the world, the population is ageing, leading to an increase in demand for healthcare. AI is seen as a potential solution to help fill workforce gaps and improve the efficiency of healthcare systems.

5. Medical research and drug discovery: AI has become a valuable tool for medical research, enabling the rapid analysis of vast genomic databases and facilitating the identification of new therapeutic targets. AI is also accelerating the drug discovery process by simulating and predicting the effects of new molecules.

6. Improved diagnosis and treatment: AI shows great potential for improving the accuracy of medical diagnoses by analysing medical images, biometric signals and patient symptoms. It can also suggest personalised treatments based on the specific characteristics of each individual.

7. Regulatory trends and investment: Regulators and healthcare stakeholders are increasingly recognising the potential of AI. They have begun to develop regulatory frameworks for its use and have invested in research and development initiatives to drive its adoption.

However, despite the promise of AI in healthcare, its integration also raises ethical questions, concerns about data privacy, and worries about the potential replacement of healthcare workers by machines. It is in this complex and dynamic context that we need to consider the future coexistence of AI and human carers, and how to make the most of this technology without compromising the quality of care and the carer-patient relationship.

The book's central question: Can artificial intelligence one day replace the carer?

At the heart of this study is a fundamental question that is arousing both enthusiasm and apprehension in the healthcare sector: is it conceivable that artificial intelligence could one day completely replace the role of the human carer?

The rapid evolution of AI in healthcare has given rise to advanced technologies capable of diagnosing diseases, analysing medical data, monitoring patients' health in real time, and even performing surgery with extreme precision. These advances have led to heated debates about whether AI could one day take on all or many of the functions currently performed by human carers.

On the one hand, proponents of this vision firmly believe that AI has the potential to surpass human capabilities in certain areas, delivering more efficient, accurate and accessible healthcare to more people. They point to AI's advantages, such as its ability to rapidly analyse large datasets, spot subtle patterns in diagnoses, and provide evidence-based treatment recommendations.

However, this perspective also raises legitimate concerns about the impact on human carers. Opponents of this vision point to the crucial role played by empathy, compassion and human contact in healthcare. They point out that the presence of a caring carer can have a therapeutic effect on patients, providing comfort and emotional support. They fear that the dehumanisation of healthcare in favour of AI could create a distance between patients and carers, thus having a negative impact on the overall quality of care.

There are also ethical concerns about liability in the event of medical errors committed by AI systems, and about the confidentiality of health data when processed by intelligent algorithms.

What's more, a fundamental question remains: even if AI can indeed perform certain specific tasks more accurately than humans, should we completely abandon human intervention in healthcare? Carers have a deep understanding of the complexity of human emotions and social interactions, which is difficult for a machine to replicate.

This book will look at these crucial issues with a critical and nuanced eye. It will explore the various aspects of integrating AI into healthcare, highlighting the benefits and challenges, while seeking to strike a balance between using AI as a tool for improvement and maintaining the importance of the human factor in healthcare. By examining available data, technological trends and ethical reflections, it will seek to provide informed perspectives on the potential role of AI as a collaborator with the human carer, while preserving the core values of the art of care.

The foundations of Artificial Intelligence in Healthcare

Definition of artificial intelligence and its applications in the healthcare sector.

Artificial intelligence (AI) is a branch of computer science that aims to create machines and systems capable of performing tasks that would normally require human intelligence. Rather than being programmed with specific instructions for each task, AI systems use sophisticated algorithms to learn from data, identify patterns and make autonomous decisions. Machine learning and deep learning are sub-fields of AI that have seen significant advances in recent years, contributing to its effectiveness in a variety of fields, including healthcare.

AI applications in the healthcare sector :

- **Medical diagnosis:** AI can analyse medical images such as X-rays, MRIs and scans to detect abnormalities with greater accuracy. It can help diagnose diseases such as cancer, heart disease, neurological conditions and many others, helping doctors to interpret results more accurately.

- **Patient forecasting and monitoring:** By analysing patient data in real time, AI can identify early warning signals and predict potential complications. This enables healthcare professionals to take preventive measures and provide more personalised care.

- **Medical record management systems:** AI makes it easier to manage and organise electronic medical records. It can extract and structure important information from records, enabling quick and easy access to patients' medical data.

- **Surgical   assistance:** AI can be used to assist surgeons during operations by providing real-time information, analysing patient data and offering advice on best surgical practice.

- **Drug discovery:** AI accelerates the drug research and development process by identifying potential therapeutic targets, simulating molecular interactions and predicting the efficacy of new chemical substances.

- **Personalised treatment:** By analysing individual patient characteristics, AI can recommend specific treatments tailored to each case, taking into account factors such as medical history, genes, and patient preferences.

- **Digital health and wellness:** AI-powered health apps, such as fitness trackers, virtual health coaches and emotional support chatbots, empower individuals to take charge of their own health and wellbeing.

Although AI applications in healthcare are promising, they are not a complete replacement for human carers. AI is often used as a tool to help healthcare professionals make informed decisions and deliver more effective care, but the human presence remains essential to provide emotional support, empathy and a deep understanding of individual patient needs. The key to successfully integrating AI into the healthcare sector lies in the harmonious collaboration between technology and human carers, harnessing the benefits of each aspect to deliver optimal patient care.

Benefits and challenges of AI in healthcare.

Benefits of AI in healthcare:

- **More accurate diagnosis:** AI can analyse vast quantities of medical data and identify subtle patterns that are often beyond human capabilities. This leads to more accurate diagnoses and early detection of disease, improving the chances of successful treatment.

- **Informed decision-making:** By providing evidence-based analysis and information, AI helps healthcare professionals make informed decisions about treatments and care plans for individual patients.

- **Continuous patient monitoring:** AI can monitor patients' vital parameters and medical data in real time, enabling any significant changes or deterioration in health to be detected quickly, facilitating early intervention.

- **Workflow optimisation:** AI can automate certain administrative and repetitive tasks, freeing up time for healthcare professionals, who can focus more on patient interaction and more complex tasks.

- **Improved medical research:** AI accelerates the discovery of new therapies and drugs by rapidly analysing vast databases and identifying potential new targets for treatment.

AI challenges in healthcare:

- **Algorithm reliability:** The reliability of AI algorithms is crucial in medicine. Misdiagnosis or inaccurate recommendations could have serious consequences for patient health. It is essential to ensure that AI systems are well trained on diverse and representative data to minimise bias.

- **Confidentiality and data security:** The use of AI in healthcare involves handling sensitive patient data. Protecting the confidentiality and security of medical data is a major challenge if unauthorised access or hacking is to be prevented.

- **Interpreting results:** The results produced by AI systems can be complex and difficult for healthcare professionals to interpret, particularly if they lack computer skills. It is crucial to develop user-friendly tools and suitable interfaces to facilitate interaction between carers and AI.

- **Patient-carer relationship:** Although AI can bring significant improvements to healthcare, it cannot replace empathy, compassion and the human relationship between patient and carer. Preserving this human dimension remains essential for high-quality, holistic care.

- **Cost and accessibility: Implementing** sophisticated AI systems can be expensive, which may make it difficult for some healthcare institutions to access them, particularly in less developed regions. Equity and accessibility of AI technologies must be key concerns to ensure that all patients benefit equitably.

In sum, the benefits of AI in healthcare are numerous and promising, offering opportunities to improve the efficiency, accuracy and personalisation of treatments. However, the technical, ethical and practical challenges must be addressed responsibly to ensure the successful integration of AI into healthcare, maximising its benefits while preserving the very essence of the carer-patient relationship.

Concrete examples of the use of AI in medicine and nursing.

- **AI-assisted medical diagnosis:** AI is increasingly being used to help doctors diagnose illnesses. For example, in medical imaging, deep learning algorithms can analyse X-rays, scans and MRIs to detect abnormalities, such as tumours, fractures or heart abnormalities. AI can also be used to help diagnose complex diseases, such as breast cancer, by identifying subtle features that might be missed by the naked eye.

- **Clinical decision support systems:** AI can be integrated into electronic medical records to provide evidence-based clinical recommendations. For example, based on patient characteristics and medical history, AI can suggest appropriate treatments, suitable drug dosages or specific preventive measures for chronic diseases.

- **Continuous patient monitoring:** AI systems can monitor the vital signs of hospitalised or intensive care patients in real time. They can detect subtle changes in vital parameters, such as blood pressure, heart rate and oxygen saturation, and alert medical staff to potentially dangerous abnormalities.

- **Surgical assistance:** AI can be used to provide real-time assistance during surgery. It can analyse live images of the surgical area to help the surgeon pinpoint anatomical structures, avoid sensitive tissue and improve the precision of surgical gestures.

- **Disease and complication prediction:** By analysing patient health data, AI can predict the risk of developing certain diseases, such as diabetes or cardiovascular disease. It can also anticipate potential complications, enabling doctors to take preventive measures to reduce the risks.

- **Health chatbots and patient monitoring:** AI-powered health chatbots can provide personalised health advice to patients, answer common medical questions, and monitor patients' health status at home. These tools can be useful for monitoring patients with chronic conditions and for providing emotional support and medical reminders.

- **Medical research and drug discovery:** AI is being used to accelerate medical research by analysing genomic databases, identifying potential therapeutic targets and predicting the efficacy of new molecules for drug development.

These examples show the extent to which AI can be used in healthcare, demonstrating its potential to improve healthcare, speed up diagnosis and treatment, and optimise clinical processes. However, it is important to note that AI is not intended to replace healthcare professionals, but rather to assist them and improve their decision-making, while preserving the importance of human interaction and empathy in patient care.

More than just a fad, artificial intelligence is now widely used in many sectors and professions. The explosion in the volume of digital data available to businesses, the computing power available and the maturity of the technologies used to process it are all factors in the tremendous growth of artificial intelligence. In this context, tedious and repetitive operations performed manually are now largely automated in order to best assist users in carrying out their various tasks. A Like other professions, such as customer relations, the healthcare sector is today one of the major beneficiaries of the many contributions made by artificial intelligence.

A practical response to strategic needs

A many levels (research, analysis, etc.), artificial intelligence is now a real ally for healthcare professionals. Used in experimental form until recently, it is now widely deployed in various use cases. Among the most concrete applications, those linked to the detection of diseases and infections are particularly relevant and are starting to become real 'must haves', especially for laboratories that have to manage large volumes of data and samples. The idea is to implement genuine diagnostic support tools.

For example, by combining imaging with artificial intelligence, doctors and staff in charge of analysing samples will be able to improve their diagnosis with the help of artificial intelligence. In cancer screening, for example, this means more reliable diagnoses and a clear reduction in misinterpretations, which can have dramatic consequences. Artificial intelligence therefore represents a formidable diagnostic aid for healthcare professionals, one that is ultra-precise, reliable and reproducible.

AI is at the heart of the medicine of the future. Diagnostic assistance, computer-assisted surgery, medical robots, predictive medicine, epidemic anticipation, patient triage, development of new treatments.

Here are 5 examples of how technology is being used in the medical sector.

1. IA TO GUIDE PATIENTS MORE EFFECTIVELY

Imagine listing your symptoms in an encyclopaedia of all existing illnesses. That's the idea that Montreal's CHUM is currently experimenting with for emergency .triage Patients arrive at A&E, enter their information into a computer and it sorts them according to their degree of urgency. The AI also determines whether the problem is respiratory, pulmonary, cardiac or other. "We are currently comparing this machine triage with human triage. The machine saves time, but we want to make sure that this triage is done wisely and that it is of high quality, because it may work well for one type of patient but not for another," explains Dr Fabrice Brunet, President and CEO of the CHUM. "We never take it for granted that, because something is new and innovative, it will be beneficial. You have to remain critical. AI, like any innovation, needs to be evaluated and measured to ensure that it is beneficial," warns Fabrice Brunet.

2. IA FOR BETTER REMOTE CONSULTATION

As with triage in hospital emergency departments, AI can be a valuable tool for guiding patients at a distance. Quebec-based telemedicine platform Dialogue implements AI to simplify the care pathway. "It's essentially a question of collecting a complete and accurate image of the patient," explains Alexis Smirnov, Dialogue's Director of Technology. For example, a patient with a skin problem might tell the chatbot ChloChloéThe chatbot may also be asked to send a photo of the problem. The data and photo are then validated by a healthcare professional. If the next step involves making an appointment with a dermatologist, the process can again be automated. In this way, the doctor simply asks the system to take the patient to the next stage of their journey. The Dialogue team makes it clear that this tool will never replace the human: "At Dialogue, we believe that AI technology is not advanced enough to make human, medically-based judgements -

particularly when you consider the human factors involved in these types of decisions. That said, however, there is a big difference between making medical decisions and optimising the non-medical components of a patient's care pathway."

3. IA TO SPEED UP DRUG DEVELOPMENT

It takes around ten years and millions of dollars before a drug is brought to market. And in the case of epidemics like Covid, the need for a pharmaceutical solution is urgent. One way of reducing vaccine development time is to optimise preclinical research. This is the objective ofInVivo AIa start-up created by three Quebec doctoral students driven by the desire to speed up the drug development process, so that medicines can be made available to patients more quickly. They have pooled their complementary expertise in molecular biology, computational neuroscience and machine learning to create a technology that streamlines pharmaceutical research and development.

"At present, the drug development process is still fairly intuitive," explains Therence Bois, co-founder of InVivo AI. "For a specific therapeutic target, a researcher tests a range of molecules, often quite randomly, and repeats the experiments until he finds one that is active for the target of interest, all in a very iterative way. The technologies ofInVivo AI technologies analyse the édata énérgenerated by these researchers and écreate èmodels that can be used to simulate these experiments computationally and get through this process more quickly."

4. IA TO IMPROVE DIAGNOSIS

With the proliferation of medical tools, doctors are having to take more and more data into account. The medical field in which AI is most present today is the interpretation of medical imaging and radiology. Certain cancers, such as lung or breast cancer, are very difficult to identify on images produced by scanners. Programmes are capable of identifying anomalies that are undetectable to the naked eye, enabling early tumours to be detected more reliably and treatments to be targeted more effectively.

Montreal start-up Imagia s mission is to speed up the detection of certain types of cancer, develop new personalised treatments and accelerate clinical research and the development of new treatments. Its Evidens platform uses the algorithms of a patented technology called Deep Radiomics to produce biomarkers (i.e. indicators that make it possible to measure normal or pathological processes linked to a therapeutic intervention) from digital images, so as to detect the appearance of an anomaly in a patient or monitor its development.

These programmes are capable of "learning by themselves", since they store all the biological anomalies detected in their memory, and are therefore more accurate with each diagnosis. In-depth, personalised treatments for each patient then become more accessible.

AI can also help detect pathologies in extremely sensitive areas. The Quebec company Diagnos has developed an AI capable of detecting diabetic retinopathy. A complication of diabetes that affects 50% of type 2 patients and is responsible for 5% of cases of blindness worldwide. Using a photo of the retina, the programme is able to detect the first signs of the disease. These photos are taken in just a few minutes using special cameras already available in a number of clinics, optometry centres and pharmacies here and abroad. The system has already analysed the eyes of almost 225,000 patients in 16 countries. André Larente, President of Diagnos, claims that the system is able to detect 98.5% of cases of retinopathy.

5 - MEDICAL ROBOTS

More and more operations are being carried out using surgical robots, tools that improve comfort for both surgeon and patient and simplify the post-operative .period Robotics is booming in the healthcare sector.

With the pandemic in China, medical robots have helped to reduce the workload in hospitals. Orion Stara robotics company supported by Cheetah Mobile, has deployed robots that have helped improve preliminary diagnosis and treatment, primary disclosure of medical information and fixed-point delivery of medical supplies in hospitals.

The current role of the carer

Description of the traditional role of the care assistant.

Healthcare assistants are essential to the smooth running of the healthcare system and the quality of services provided to patients. Their role is primarily focused on assisting and supporting patients in their daily lives, as well as supporting other members of the medical team. Here are the main characteristics of the traditional role of the healthcare assistant:

- **Basic patient care:** The care assistant is responsible for providing basic care to patients, such as personal hygiene (grooming, bathing, dressing), changing bed linen, helping with mobility, and assisting with elimination needs.

- **Patient monitoring:** Healthcare assistants regularly monitor patients' state of health, noting and reporting any significant variations or changes. They may take temperatures, measure blood pressure and observe vital signs to detect any deterioration in the patient's condition.

- **Emotional support:** A crucial aspect of the care assistant's role is to provide emotional support to patients. This may involve listening to their concerns, responding to their emotional needs, and creating a reassuring and caring environment.

- **Assistance with daily activities:** The care assistant helps patients with their daily activities, such as eating, getting around and leisure activities. They ensure that patients feel comfortable and supported in their daily routine.

- **Working with the care team:** Healthcare assistants work closely with nurses, doctors and other healthcare professionals. They pass on important information about patients, take part in team meetings and help to coordinate care.

- **Records management and reporting:** Healthcare assistants may be responsible for keeping patient records up to date, noting down important observations and writing reports on patients' state of health.

- **Risk prevention:** Healthcare assistants are alert to the risks of falls, bedsores and infections among patients. They take preventive measures to reduce these risks and ensure the safety of patients in their environment.

- **Communication with families:** The nursing auxiliary may be in direct contact with patients' families to inform them of the progress of their state of health, answer their questions and provide them with support at this difficult time.

- **Compliance with hygiene and safety standards:** Healthcare assistants must comply with hygiene and safety protocols to prevent the spread of infections and ensure a clean and safe environment for patients.

The role of the healthcare assistant is characterised by a strong commitment to the well-being of patients and a holistic approach to care. By providing essential care and creating meaningful links with patients, the carer plays a central role in the humanisation of healthcare and contributes to the recovery and overall well-being of the individuals under their care.

- Personal accounts and experiences of the author as a care assistant for 15 years.

As an experienced care assistant who has practised for many years, I have witnessed many emotionally charged experiences, moments of joy, sadness and unique challenges in the field of healthcare. Here are some of the personal stories and experiences that have shaped my career:

- **The importance of empathy and compassion: Over the** years, I've learned that empathy and compassion are essential qualities for creating a meaningful bond with patients. In my testimonials, I describe how a simple attentive listening ear, a word of encouragement or a kind gesture can make all the difference to an anxious or suffering patient. These moments of humanity have often been a source of comfort to patients and their families.

- **The power of resilience in patients:** I've been lucky enough to accompany patients on their healing journey, which has allowed me to bear witness to the remarkable resilience of individuals in the face of adversity. I share inspiring stories of patients who, despite difficult medical conditions, have found the strength to fight, overcome obstacles and regain quality of life.

- **The weight of goodbyes:** Working in the healthcare sector, I've had to deal with some heartbreaking moments, including saying goodbye to patients who have succumbed to their illnesses. These experiences had a profound effect on me and strengthened my desire to provide compassionate care and support to patients right up to their final moments.

- **The evolution of medical technologies:** I have witnessed the increasing introduction of medical technologies and AI in healthcare. In my experiences, I share how these technological advances have sometimes simplified certain clinical tasks, but have also raised questions about the impact on the patient-carer relationship.

- **Workload challenges:** Often working in demanding care environments, I've had to deal with the challenges associated with high workloads. I share experiences where I have had to juggle various responsibilities and provide quality care despite limited resources.

- **Patient gratitude:** I remember the times when patients or their relatives expressed their gratitude for my care and dedication. These expressions of gratitude have been a source of motivation and personal satisfaction in my professional career.

In recounting these stories and experiences, I offer an intimate insight into the complex reality of working as a healthcare assistant, my highs and lows, and the emotions that accompany this essential profession. These stories reflect the author's deep commitment to patient-centred care and highlight the continuing importance of the human factor in healthcare.

The importance of empathy and communication in the carer-patient relationship.

Empathy and communication play a crucial role in the carer-patient relationship. They are essential for establishing a bond of trust, understanding the patient's needs and providing high-quality, person-centred care. Here's how important these elements are in the carer-patient relationship:

1. Creating an environment of trust: Empathy shows that the carer understands and feels the patient's emotions, which builds trust. Patients are more likely to feel comfortable and secure when they know that their carer understands and supports them emotionally.

2. Understanding the patient's needs : Empathy enables carers to put themselves in the patient's shoes, to perceive their concerns, fears and worries. This helps to provide personalised care that takes account of the patient's values, beliefs and preferences.

3. Encouraging the expression of emotions: When patients are faced with health challenges, they may experience a wide range of emotions, including fear, anxiety and sadness. Empathetic communication encourages patients to express their emotions, which can help to improve their psychological well-being.

4. Improved therapeutic compliance: Empathetic communication enables the carer to better explain treatments and medical instructions in a way that the patient can understand. This increases the chances that the patient will follow the recommended care plan correctly.

5. More effective diagnosis: Empathy promotes better communication between patient and carer, making it easier to gather important medical information. A patient who feels listened to is more likely to provide precise details of their symptoms, which can lead to a more accurate and rapid diagnosis.

6. Reducing stress and anxiety: For patients facing health problems, emotional support can have a soothing and comforting effect. Empathy and caring communication can help reduce the stress and anxiety associated with medical care.

7. Improved patient satisfaction: Patients feel better cared for and satisfied when carers give them empathetic attention. Warm and respectful communication can improve their overall healthcare experience.

8. Strengthening the therapeutic relationship: Empathetic communication fosters a solid therapeutic relationship between patient and carer. It creates an environment in which the patient feels heard and respected, which facilitates collaboration in the healing process.

In short, empathy and communication are fundamental pillars of the carer-patient relationship. They foster a holistic approach to care and help to establish a bond of trust that is essential to providing quality care, centred on patients' individual needs and preferences. Integrating these qualities into the practice of care providers helps to humanise healthcare and promote the overall well-being of patients.

Artificial Intelligence
as a Caregiver's Assistant

Analysis of AI as a tool for improving carers' tasks.

Artificial intelligence (AI) can play an essential role as a tool for improving the tasks of healthcare workers. It offers unique capabilities that can enhance the efficiency, accuracy and quality of care provided. Here is an in-depth look at how AI can be used to support and improve the work of caregivers:

1. AI-assisted diagnosis: AI can rapidly analyse vast quantities of medical data, such as medical images, laboratory analyses and electronic health records. By helping to identify subtle patterns, AI can provide additional information to assist healthcare professionals in diagnosis and medical decision-making.

2. Predicting complications and risks: By analysing patient health data, AI can anticipate potential complications and individual risks. This enables carers to implement tailored preventive strategies to improve patient outcomes and reduce avoidable hospitalisations.

3. Patient monitoring and real-time response: AI systems can monitor patients' vital parameters in real time, flag up abnormal variations and alert carers in an emergency. This enables rapid intervention and can save lives in critical situations.

4. Workflow optimisation: AI can automate certain administrative tasks, such as scheduling appointments, managing files and billing. By freeing up valuable time for carers, they can focus more on patient interaction and more clinical aspects.

5. Assistance with drug prescribing: AI can help detect potentially dangerous drug interactions and suggest dose adjustments to avoid prescribing errors. This reduces the risk of medical errors and improves patient safety.

6. Personalised treatment plans: By analysing patient health data, AI can recommend specific treatments tailored to each individual, taking into account factors such as medical history, genetic characteristics and patient preferences.

7. Emotional support for patients: AI can be used to develop emotional support chatbots that interact with patients to provide psychological support and answer their questions. This can help improve patients' emotional wellbeing and increase their engagement in their own healing process.

However, despite these benefits, it is important to note that AI cannot completely replace the expertise and empathy of human carers. Healthcare is deeply rooted in the human aspect, and interaction with a caring carer can have a significant impact on patient recovery and satisfaction.

Therefore, the successful integration of AI as a tool to improve caregivers' tasks must be done in a balanced way, preserving the importance of the human factor in healthcare. AI should be seen as a collaborative partner, enabling carers to make more informed decisions and deliver higher quality care, while continuing to foster a patient-centred approach and promote a trusting relationship between patient and carer.

How AI can help in diagnosis, patient monitoring, medical records management, etc.

How AI can help in diagnosis, patient monitoring, medical records management, etc.

Artificial intelligence (AI) has enormous potential to transform and improve various aspects of healthcare. Here's how it can benefit diagnosis, patient monitoring, medical records management and other areas:

1. AI-assisted diagnosis: AI can analyse large amounts of medical data, including medical images, laboratory test results and electronic health records, to help doctors make more accurate diagnoses. AI algorithms can spot subtle anomalies in medical images, which can lead to early detection of diseases such as cancer and cardiovascular conditions.

2. Real-time patient monitoring: AI systems can continuously monitor the vital signs of patients in hospital or intensive care. They detect significant changes in physiological parameters such as heart rate, blood pressure and oxygen saturation, and alert healthcare professionals to any abnormalities, enabling early intervention in the event of an emergency.

3. Predicting and managing complications: By analysing patient health data, AI can predict the risk of developing certain medical complications, such as hospital-acquired infections or blood clots. This enables healthcare professionals to take targeted preventive measures to reduce these risks and improve patient outcomes.

4. Medical record management: AI facilitates the management of electronic medical records by automating certain tasks, such as extracting and structuring relevant information from records. This enables doctors and nurses to access important medical data more quickly and make informed decisions.

5. Surgical assistance: AI can be used to provide real-time assistance during surgery. It can analyse live images and provide useful information to the surgeon, improving precision and reducing the risk of error.

6. Disease detection and prevention: AI can be used to analyse patients' risk factors, medical history and genetic data to help them adopt preventive health behaviours. This can lead to earlier detection of disease and better management of chronic conditions.

7. Treatment recommendation systems: AI can analyse clinical data from similar patients to recommend effective treatments. These personalised recommendation systems can help doctors choose the best treatment for each patient, taking into account individual factors.

8. Clinical decision support: AI can provide evidence-based information to help healthcare professionals make informed decisions. By integrating current medical knowledge and evidence, AI systems can help formulate more effective treatment plans.

However, it is important to stress that despite all these benefits, AI should not replace the skill, empathy and clinical judgement of healthcare professionals. The integration of AI into healthcare needs to be done in a balanced way, using AI as an assistive tool to support carers and improve care while preserving the importance of human interaction and the trusting relationship between patient and carer.

Future prospects for AI as a "colleague" of the carer.

The future prospects for artificial intelligence (AI) as a 'colleague' to the carer are promising and exciting. AI will continue to evolve and play an increasingly significant role in healthcare, collaborating with carers to improve the quality of care and efficiency of medical services. Here are some future prospects for this relationship between AI and the carer:

1. Advanced clinical assistance: With continued advances in machine learning and natural language processing, AI will be able to provide even more sophisticated clinical assistance. It will be able to interact with carers in a more contextual and personalised way, providing evidence-based recommendations for diagnoses, treatments and care plans.

2. Prevention and early detection of disease: AI will continue to play a key role in the prevention and early detection of disease. AI algorithms will become increasingly effective at analysing patients' medical data, enabling risk factors to be identified and early signs of disease to be detected, improving the chances of successful treatment.

3. Precision medicine: AI will enable treatments to be better targeted to the specific characteristics of each patient, leading to more advanced precision medicine. AI models will be able to predict how a patient will react to a specific treatment, helping to choose the most effective treatments with fewer side effects.

4. Medical robotics: In collaboration with medical robots, AI can be used to perform more precise and less invasive surgical procedures. Robots can be equipped with AI to help surgeons perform more complex procedures with greater precision.

5. Enhanced healthcare chatbots: AI-powered chatbots will continue to develop as patient support tools. They will be able to answer a wider range of medical questions, provide more personalised health advice and monitor patients' health at home.

6. Medical training and decision-making: AI could be used in medical training programmes to simulate complex clinical cases and help future carers to develop their diagnostic and decision-making skills. Caregivers will also be able to access medical knowledge bases that are constantly updated thanks to AI.

7. Improved efficiency of care: By automating certain administrative and repetitive tasks, AI will free up time for carers, allowing them to focus more on direct patient care and more complex clinical tasks.

However, with these opportunities also come challenges. It will be essential to ensure the security and privacy of patient data, mitigate potential biases in AI algorithms and ensure that the integration of AI into healthcare is ethical and patient-centric.

Ultimately, the increasing integration of AI as a carer's 'colleague' has the potential to dramatically improve healthcare, making diagnoses more accurate and treatments more personalised, while preserving the importance of the carer-patient relationship and the human factor in healthcare.

Ethical and legal challenges

Discussion of the ethical dilemmas associated with the use of AI in healthcare.

The increasing integration of artificial intelligence (AI) into healthcare raises many complex ethical dilemmas. While AI can offer significant benefits, it also raises concerns about data privacy, accountability, autonomous decision-making and trust in healthcare. Here are some of the most important ethical dilemmas related to the use of AI in healthcare:

1. Data confidentiality and privacy: AI requires access to vast amounts of medical data to operate effectively. This raises concerns about the confidentiality of patients' medical information and the protection of their privacy. It is crucial that robust security measures are put in place to prevent data breaches and ensure that patients' personal information is protected.

2. Algorithmic biases: AI algorithms are trained on historical datasets, which may contain systemic biases based on factors such as age, gender, race or ethnicity. This can lead to inequalities in diagnosis, treatment and health outcomes. Monitoring and reducing bias in AI models is essential to ensure fair and non-discriminatory care.

3. Responsibility and autonomous decision-making: When AI takes over certain clinical tasks, responsibility for healthcare decisions can be diluted between the algorithm and the healthcare professional. In the event of an error or problem, it can be difficult to determine who is responsible. Healthcare professionals will always need to play an active role in decision-making, and responsibility will need to be clearly established in the event of adverse events.

4. Lack of empathy and human communication: AI can provide data-driven answers and recommendations, but it cannot replace empathy and human communication. Patients need interaction with compassionate and caring carers to feel understood and emotionally supported. It is therefore essential to strike a balance between using AI to improve care and maintaining a human approach in the carer-patient relationship.

5. Patient autonomy: AI can provide personalised treatment recommendations, but this can also raise questions about patient autonomy. Some patients may feel disempowered if treatment choices are heavily influenced by algorithms. It is important to allow patients to participate actively in decisions about their health and treatment.

6. Inequalities in access to AI technologies: AI technologies can be expensive to implement and maintain. This can lead to inequalities in access to advanced AI-based healthcare, particularly in disadvantaged regions or communities. It is crucial to ensure that AI does not widen the gap between patients and that it is used in an equitable and inclusive way.

In sum, the use of AI in healthcare offers exciting opportunities to improve care, diagnostic accuracy and treatment effectiveness. However, resolving the ethical dilemmas associated with AI is essential to ensuring fair, transparent and patient-centred care. Consideration of ethical issues from the outset and responsible use of AI are essential to maximise its benefits while minimising its potential risks.

Protecting patient privacy and securing health data.

Protecting patient privacy and securing healthcare data are key concerns when using artificial intelligence (AI) in healthcare. Medical data is extremely sensitive, containing confidential personal and medical information about patients. Here are some key measures to ensure the privacy and security of health data in the context of AI in healthcare:

1. Informed consent: Before collecting, processing or using patient data, it is essential to obtain informed consent from patients. Patients must be informed in a clear and transparent way about how their data will be used, why it is needed and how it will be protected.

2. Anonymisation and pseudonymisation of data: Before being used to train AI algorithms, medical data can be anonymised or pseudonymised to avoid direct identification of patients. This considerably reduces the risk of inadvertent disclosure of sensitive data.

3. Data encryption : Healthcare data must be stored and transmitted securely using robust encryption protocols. This prevents any unauthorised person from accessing sensitive information in the event of a breach or intrusion.

4. Restricted access and access control: Health professionals and researchers who use health data must have restricted access only to the information necessary for their specific tasks. Strict access control must be in place to ensure that only authorised persons can access the data.

5. Device and network security: The devices and networks used to store and process healthcare data must be secure and protected against computer attacks. Regular updates, firewalls and anti-virus software are essential to prevent security breaches.

6. Training and awareness: Regular training of medical staff and healthcare professionals on best practice in data protection and IT security is essential. Raising awareness of security risks helps to minimise the human errors that can lead to data breaches.

7. Regulatory Compliance: Healthcare AI systems must comply with data protection and privacy laws and regulations, such as the General Data Protection Regulation (GDPR) in Europe or HIPAA regulations in the US.

8. Monitoring and auditing: Continuous monitoring and regular audits must be carried out to detect anomalies and suspicious activities, thus ensuring a rapid response in the event of a security breach.
By implementing these measures, healthcare institutions and providers can strengthen the protection of patient privacy and ensure the security of health data when using AI. The aim is to ensure that the benefits of AI in healthcare are achieved without compromising the public's trust in the security and confidentiality of their medical information.

Liability for AI errors or misinterpretations.

Liability for artificial intelligence (AI) errors or misinterpretations is a complex and crucial topic to address when AI is used in healthcare. As AI increasingly makes clinical decisions and provides medical recommendations, it is important to determine who is liable in the event of an error or adverse outcome. Here are some key aspects of liability related to AI in healthcare:

1. Shared responsibility: Responsibility for healthcare involving AI must be shared between the AI itself, the developers of the algorithm, the manufacturers of the AI system and the healthcare professionals using the AI. Each party must assume its share of responsibility according to its role and actions.

2. AI developers: The designers and developers of AI algorithms have a responsibility to create reliable and safe models. This means implementing rigorous testing, identifying and mitigating potential biases, and ensuring that AI operates transparently and in compliance with ethical and regulatory standards.

3. AI system manufacturers: AI system manufacturers must guarantee the reliability, safety and compliance of their products. They must also provide regular updates to correct errors and discovered vulnerabilities.

4. Healthcare professionals: Healthcare professionals using AI have a responsibility to understand the limitations of AI, to validate the results provided by AI and to make informed decisions based on their clinical expertise. They must also report any problems or unexpected results related to the use of AI.

5. Transparency and explanation: AI must be transparent in how it works and how it arrives at its conclusions. AI's decision-making mechanisms must be understandable to healthcare professionals so that they can correctly interpret the results and make informed decisions.

6. Insurance and error coverage: When AI is used to make medical decisions, it is important to have appropriate insurance policies in place to cover errors or adverse outcomes that may occur as a result of the use of AI.

7. Transparency in the use of AI: Healthcare institutions and providers must be transparent with patients about the use of AI in their care. Patients should be informed when AI is involved in their diagnosis or treatment, and they should be able to ask questions about its role in their medical care.

Liability for errors or misinterpretations of AI is a constantly evolving area. It is essential to develop clear guidelines and policies to clarify the roles and responsibilities of each party involved in the use of AI in healthcare. A collaborative approach involving AI developers, healthcare professionals, regulators and patients is needed to ensure that AI is used responsibly and safely, while maximising its benefits to improve healthcare.

Towards Harmonious Coexistence

Reflecting on the benefits of AI and human carers working together.

The cohabitation of artificial intelligence (AI) and the human carer offers a multitude of benefits that can positively transform the field of healthcare. Rather than completely replacing the human carer, AI can be used as a complementary tool to enhance the capabilities and performance of the carer. Here is a reflection on the benefits of this cohabitation:

1. Increased accuracy and efficiency: AI can analyse large amounts of medical data in record time, helping carers to obtain accurate information and make informed decisions. This can lead to more accurate diagnoses, personalised treatment plans and more efficient care management.

2. Early detection of disease: AI can help identify early signs of disease or potential complications by analysing patient data. This enables early detection, which is crucial for improving the chances of recovery and preventing the progression of certain diseases.

3. Improved decision-making: AI can provide evidence-based information to carers, enabling them to make more informed and educated decisions. This strengthens their clinical expertise and improves the overall quality of care provided.

4. Automation of repetitive tasks: AI can take over certain administrative and repetitive tasks, allowing carers to concentrate more on interacting with patients and on the more clinical aspects of treatment.

5. Emotional support and empathy: Although AI cannot express emotions, it can be used to provide basic emotional support to patients, for example, by informing them about their state of health, answering their questions or reminding them to take their medication. This can ease the emotional burden on care staff and improve the overall patient experience.

6. Training and education: AI can be used in medical training programmes to simulate complex clinical scenarios, helping students and carers to develop their skills and expertise.

7. Care monitoring and management: AI can monitor patients' vital signs and health data in real time, enabling proactive care management and rapid intervention when needed.

8. Precision medicine: AI can be used to analyse patients' genetic and clinical data to provide more targeted and personalised treatments.

By combining the strengths of AI and the human carer, it is possible to significantly improve the quality, efficiency and accessibility of healthcare. AI can free up time and resources for carers, allowing them to focus on more complex and relational aspects of care. Ultimately, the cohabitation of AI and the human carer can contribute to more efficient, accurate and patient-centred healthcare, while preserving the very essence of the carer-patient relationship and the importance of humanity in healthcare.

The importance of emotional intelligence and human skills in healthcare.

Emotional intelligence and human skills play a fundamental and irreplaceable role in healthcare. While artificial intelligence (AI) offers advanced technological capabilities, it cannot replace the human and emotional dimension that is essential in the carer-patient relationship. Here is the importance of emotional intelligence and human skills in healthcare:

1. Empathy and understanding: Empathy is the ability to put oneself in the patient's shoes, to understand their emotions, fears and concerns. Caregivers with emotional intelligence can establish a deep connection with their patients, fostering a climate of trust and mutual understanding.

2. Emotional support: Patients may experience moments of vulnerability, fear or sadness. The presence of a warm, caring carer can provide emotional comfort and improve the patient's overall well-being.

3. Effective communication: Communication is an essential pillar of healthcare. Caregivers with high emotional intelligence can communicate with compassion and clarity, enabling them to better inform patients about their condition, treatments and decisions.

4. Relationship of trust: Human skills and emotional intelligence are at the heart of building a relationship of trust between carer and patient. This trust facilitates the patient's cooperation and adherence to the treatment plan, which in turn improves health outcomes.

5. Stress and bereavement management: At difficult times, such as a serious diagnosis or bereavement, the human skills of the carer are crucial in providing emotional support to patients and their families.

6. Adaptability to individual needs: Every patient is unique, with their own life experiences and preferences.

Emotionally intelligent carers can adapt to each patient's individual needs and personalise their approach to care.

7. Ethical decision-making: Human skills help carers to approach ethical dilemmas in a thoughtful way and to make decisions based on the patient's well-being and respect for his or her values.

8. Conflict and tension management: Conflict and tension management skills enable carers to handle stressful situations calmly and professionally.

In summary, emotional intelligence and human skills are essential in healthcare, as they promote a patient-centred approach based on compassion, empathy and understanding. As AI continues to evolve and integrate into healthcare, it is essential to recognise that the warm, human presence of carers will remain irreplaceable in delivering comprehensive, caring and holistic care. The harmonious cohabitation of AI and human skills is the key to ensuring high-quality, patient-centred healthcare tailored to individual needs.

Proposals for the successful integration of AI into existing care practices.

For the successful integration of artificial intelligence (AI) into existing healthcare practices, it is essential to follow certain proposals and best practices. Here are some ideas for the successful integration of AI into healthcare:

1. Training of healthcare professionals: Adequate training of healthcare professionals in the use of AI is essential. They need to understand how to interact with AI, interpret its results and make informed decisions based on the information provided by AI.

2. Collaboration between AI and healthcare professionals: It is important to promote a culture of collaboration between AI and healthcare professionals. AI should not be seen as a separate entity, but rather as a tool to support carers in their decisions and practice.

3. Validation and transparency: AI models used in healthcare must be rigorously validated to ensure their accuracy and reliability. In addition, transparency is essential to enable healthcare professionals to understand how AI makes decisions and to trust its results.

4. Gradual integration: Integrating AI into existing healthcare practices should be done gradually and incrementally. Starting with simple, well-defined use cases allows healthcare professionals to get used to using AI before adopting more complex applications.

5. Respect for ethics and confidentiality: It is essential to comply with ethical and regulatory standards in terms of data protection and patient confidentiality. Health data must be stored and processed securely, and patients must be informed about the use of AI in their medical care.

6. Continuous performance evaluation: It is important to continuously monitor AI performance and make adjustments based on feedback from healthcare professionals and clinical outcomes. AI must evolve in line with the changing needs and requirements of care practices.

7. Patient-centred approach: AI integration should always be patient-centric. The primary objective should be to improve health outcomes and the overall patient experience. Healthcare must remain human-centred, taking into account the individual needs and preferences of each patient.

8. Collaboration with AI developers: Healthcare professionals need to work closely with AI developers to provide feedback on specific clinical needs and desired improvements. This collaboration ensures that AI truly meets the needs of caregivers and patients.

By following these proposals, the integration of AI into existing care practices can be successful. AI can be used responsibly and effectively to improve healthcare, while preserving the importance of emotional intelligence and human skills in the carer-patient relationship. The harmonious cohabitation of AI and human caregivers is the key to providing superior healthcare, based on advanced technology and human compassion.

En Route to the Future

Projections on the evolution of AI in healthcare.

Projections for the evolution of artificial intelligence (AI) in healthcare are promising and point to a future full of possibilities. Here are some projections of how AI could evolve in healthcare:

1. Advanced precision medicine: AI will continue to improve precision medicine by analysing massive datasets, such as the patient's genome, medical history and laboratory data. This will enable better targeting of treatments and personalised care for each individual.

2. Early diagnosis of diseases: Thanks to machine learning and the analysis of medical images, AI will be able to detect the precursors of diseases at an early stage, enabling faster and more effective treatment.

3. More advanced medical robots: AI-enabled medical robots will continue to develop and assist surgeons in more complex interventions, reducing risks and improving the accuracy of surgical procedures.

4. Smart health systems: Hospitals and health centres could adopt AI-based smart health systems to improve patient management, resource planning, workflow optimisation and clinical decision-making.

5. Advanced healthcare chatbots: Healthcare chatbots will become more sophisticated, able to provide more precise and personalised answers to patients' medical questions, offering additional out-of-hours support.

6. Revolution in medical research: AI will accelerate medical research by rapidly analysing vast data sets to identify new drugs, innovative treatments and promising avenues for curing certain diseases.

7. Epidemic prevention: AI will be used to monitor epidemiological data in real time and prevent the spread of infectious diseases by quickly identifying outbreaks and taking preventive measures.

8. Clinical decision support systems: AI-based clinical decision support systems will be widely used to provide real-time recommendations to healthcare professionals when making complex clinical decisions.

9. Advanced analysis of health data: AI will enable more advanced analysis of health data, identifying previously unnoticed trends and risk factors, paving the way for new preventive and therapeutic approaches.

10. Seamless integration of AI: Over time, AI will integrate more seamlessly into healthcare practices, becoming an integral part of healthcare professionals' workflow, without disrupting the caregiver-patient relationship.

However, it is important to recognise that the evolution of AI in healthcare will also require continued reflection on ethical issues, data security, accountability and fairness. It is essential to ensure that the integration of AI is done in a responsible, patient-centred way and in collaboration with healthcare professionals, in order to maximise the benefits of this technology while minimising the potential risks.

Which functions could be fully automated, and which tasks will still require a human presence?

Some healthcare functions could be fully automated thanks to artificial intelligence (AI) and robotics, while other tasks will always require a human presence. Here are some examples of functions that can be automated and tasks that will always require human presence and intervention:

Functions that can be automated :
- **Medical imaging analysis:** AI can analyse medical images, such as X-rays, MRIs and scans, to detect anomalies or pathologies.

- **Health data analysis:** AI can process and analyse vast quantities of health data to identify trends, risk factors and correlations.
- **Medical records management:** AI systems can be used to manage and organise patients' medical records more efficiently.

- **Assistance with medical prescriptions:** AI can recommend appropriate treatments or medicines based on the patient's medical history and available data.

- **Patient monitoring:** AI devices can monitor patients' vital signs in real time and alert medical staff to any abnormalities.

- **Patient triage:** AI can help triage patients according to the severity of their condition and prioritise care.

Tasks requiring a human presence :
- **The carer-patient relationship:** The human relationship between carer and patient is essential for

building trust, offering emotional support and providing holistic care.

- **Complex diagnosis:** Complex diagnoses and unusual clinical situations require the expertise and intuition of a qualified healthcare professional.

- **Empathetic communication:** Empathetic communication and understanding of the patient's emotions cannot be replaced by automated systems.

- **Ethical decision-making:** Ethical dilemmas in healthcare require human reflection and decision-making, taking into account the patient's values and preferences.

- **Care coordination:** Coordination between the various members of the care team and overall treatment planning require organisational and relational skills specific to healthcare professionals.

- **Palliative and end-of-life care:** Palliative care and end-of-life discussions require a compassionate human presence and a sensitive approach to supporting patients and their families.

- **Training and education:** Teaching, training and mentoring future healthcare professionals requires human interaction and expertise.

In short, artificial intelligence has the potential to transform many functions and tasks in healthcare by improving the efficiency and accuracy of diagnosis and treatment. However, the human presence will remain essential for the emotional, ethical and relational aspects of healthcare, ensuring that patients receive comprehensive, human-centred care that respects their individual needs. The key lies in a harmonious cohabitation between the technological advances of AI and the human skills of healthcare professionals.

Potential impact on healthcare training and professional development.

The increasing integration of artificial intelligence (AI) into healthcare will have a significant impact on healthcare training and the evolution of the medical professions. Here are some key points about this potential impact:

1. More training on AI and technology: Healthcare training programmes will need to incorporate more teaching on AI, machine learning, data analysis and medical technology. Future healthcare professionals will need to be familiar with these tools to effectively use AI in their practice.

2. Adapting training programmes: Training programmes in medicine, nursing and other areas of healthcare will need to be adapted to include specific AI-related skills, such as interpreting AI results, working with clinical decision support systems and managing smart medical technologies.

3. Development of new specialties: The emergence of AI in healthcare could give rise to new specialties, such as medical AI experts, health data analysis specialists and healthcare professionals specialising in integrating AI into care.

4. Need for additional skills: Future healthcare professionals will need to develop additional skills, such as understanding AI algorithms, health data ethics and the ability to work collaboratively with automated systems.

5. Redefinition of traditional roles: With the automation of certain tasks, the traditional roles of healthcare professionals could evolve. For example, carers could focus more on the emotional and relational aspects of care, while AI would take over certain administrative and analytical tasks.

6. Ongoing training: Practising healthcare professionals will also need to undergo ongoing training to keep up to date with technological advances in AI and to develop the skills needed to use it effectively.

7. Development of new data management skills: With AI, the amount of data generated in healthcare will increase dramatically. Healthcare professionals will need to acquire skills in data management, privacy protection and information security to manage these massive data flows responsibly.

8. Interdisciplinary collaboration: AI will require closer collaboration between healthcare professionals and experts in computer science, artificial intelligence and data science. Care teams could include AI specialists working hand-in-hand with doctors and nurses.

In sum, the integration of AI into healthcare will lead to an evolution of medical professions and healthcare training. The acquisition of new skills related to AI and technology, as well as the development of emerging specialties, will be necessary to enable healthcare professionals to take full advantage of the benefits of AI while preserving the importance of emotional intelligence and human skills in the healthcare-patient relationship. Ongoing training and adaptability will be key to making a success of this transition to AI-enhanced medical practice.

Towards predictive medicine: How AI anticipates individual health needs

The emergence of predictive medicine

The emergence of predictive medicine marks an important step in the evolution of modern medicine. Predictive medicine involves using clinical, genetic and environmental data to identify potential risks of developing certain diseases or medical conditions in an individual. Thanks to advances in artificial intelligence and machine learning, predictive medicine has become a reality, transforming the way healthcare professionals approach disease prevention and management.

Advances in the collection and analysis of large amounts of medical data have opened up new opportunities to anticipate the risk of disease even before symptoms appear. Predictive medicine relies on the ability of AI to extract valuable information from large datasets, including medical history, lifestyle habits, genetic factors and environmental data. This data is then used to assess an individual's risk of developing certain diseases, such as heart disease, diabetes, cancer, neurodegenerative diseases and many others.

The practical applications of predictive medicine are numerous. For example, AI can be used to analyse the results of genetic tests and predict the risk of developing hereditary diseases. Similarly, it can help identify specific risk factors for a given patient, taking into account their genetic profile and medical history, in order to propose personalised preventive measures and tailored treatment plans.

By enabling early detection of the risk of disease, predictive medicine offers numerous advantages for patients and healthcare professionals alike. It makes it possible to target medical interventions more accurately, prevent the onset of potentially serious illnesses and encourage a preventive approach to health. What's more, by identifying high-risk individuals, predictive medicine can help reduce healthcare costs by avoiding costly treatments and reducing hospital admissions.

However, the emergence of predictive medicine also raises important ethical and social issues. The confidentiality of genetic and medical data is a crucial issue, as the disclosure of such information could have implications for privacy and potential discrimination. In addition, equitable access to predictive medicine must be guaranteed to avoid any exacerbation of health inequalities.

In conclusion, the emergence of predictive medicine represents a major advance in healthcare. Thanks to the use of AI to analyse and exploit medical data, predictive medicine offers new prospects for a proactive approach to health, by identifying the risks of diseases before they manifest themselves clinically. However, responsible implementation of predictive medicine is essential, taking into account ethical considerations, privacy protection and equity in access to predictive healthcare.

Big data and machine learning

Big data and machine learning are two key concepts that have contributed significantly to the emergence of artificial intelligence (AI) and its applications in various fields, including health.

The term 'big data' refers to the massive collection of data, often of great variety and velocity, from a variety of sources such as electronic medical records, medical monitoring devices, wearable sensors, clinical studies, scientific publications, social networks and many others. This data is generally of such high volume that it exceeds the capacity of traditional data management tools to store, process and analyse it effectively. This is where 'big data' comes in, providing methods and technologies to manipulate, analyse and derive meaningful information from these vast data sets.

Machine learning is a branch of AI that enables machines to learn from data without being explicitly programmed. Rather than following specific instructions, machine learning algorithms use data to identify patterns, relationships and trends, and then apply this knowledge to make predictions or decisions. Machine learning is particularly powerful when used with large amounts of data, as it can uncover complex patterns and hidden information that would be difficult to detect by traditional means.

In the field of healthcare, the combined use of big data and machine learning has had a considerable impact. AI systems can process massive amounts of medical data to identify patterns of behaviour and responses to treatment. For example, big data analysis combined with machine learning can help predict an individual's risk of developing certain diseases based on their genetic characteristics, medical history and lifestyle habits.

In addition, Big Data makes it possible to create centralised, interconnected medical databases that can be used for epidemiological studies and large-scale clinical research. It also facilitates the implementation of evidence-based preventive medicine programmes, enabling personalised, early treatment of health problems.

However, the use of big data and machine learning in medicine also raises significant challenges, particularly in terms of privacy, data security and algorithmic bias. It is essential to ensure that medical data is handled ethically and securely, and that machine learning algorithms are rigorously validated to avoid discrimination or misinterpretation of results.

In conclusion, the marriage of big data and machine learning has transformed the way medicine is practised. These technologies make it possible to extract meaningful information from vast sets of medical data, opening up new prospects for predictive medicine, biomedical research and improving the quality of healthcare. However, their use must be accompanied by ethical and responsible reflection to ensure their successful and beneficial integration into the healthcare field.

Predicting genetic diseases

Predicting genetic diseases is one of the most promising areas of predictive medicine, made possible by advances in genomics and artificial intelligence. This approach aims to use an individual's genetic information to identify the risk of developing certain hereditary diseases even before clinical symptoms appear.

The study of the human genome has revealed that many diseases have a genetic component that can predispose certain individuals to developing them. Variations in genes can influence an individual's susceptibility to a specific disease, and certain genetic mutations can be strongly associated with certain pathologies.

Technological advances in genome sequencing have enabled faster and more cost-effective analysis of an individual's genes. Next-generation sequencers can analyse a patient's DNA to identify genetic variants that may be associated with specific diseases. However, interpreting this complex genomic data requires sophisticated computational approaches, which is where artificial intelligence, particularly machine learning, comes in.

Machine learning algorithms can analyse large sets of genomic data and health profiles to identify patterns and associations between specific genetic variations and particular diseases. By combining this information with additional medical data such as family medical history, lifestyle and environment, it becomes possible to predict the risk of developing a genetic disease with greater accuracy.

The prediction of genetic diseases can have major implications for public and individual health. It can enable early identification of individuals at high risk, opening up opportunities for increased surveillance, preventive measures and appropriate medical interventions. It can also help families to make informed decisions about family planning and preconception genetic testing.

However, it is essential to consider the ethical and social issues associated with the prediction of genetic diseases. Disclosure of genetic disease risks can raise concerns about stigma, insurance and employment discrimination, as well as issues of confidentiality and informed consent. It is therefore crucial to ensure an ethical and responsible approach to the use of genetic disease prediction, guaranteeing respect for patient privacy and providing adequate support for the interpretation of results.

In conclusion, the prediction of genetic diseases is a promising application of predictive medicine, made possible by the integration of genomic sequencing and artificial intelligence. This approach offers the potential for early identification of the risk of hereditary diseases and personalised care for patients. However, ethical considerations must be taken into account to ensure that this technology is used responsibly, beneficially and fairly in healthcare.

Clinical decision support systems

Clinical Decision Support Systems (CDSS) are sophisticated IT tools that use artificial intelligence and data processing technologies to support healthcare professionals in their clinical decision-making. These systems aim to provide doctors, nurses and other healthcare professionals with valuable information and recommendations based on sound medical evidence, in order to improve the quality of care and patient outcomes.

CFDS uses sophisticated algorithms to analyse large amounts of medical data from a variety of sources, such as electronic medical records, laboratory results, medical images, clinical research and treatment protocols. By integrating this data, CFs can provide faster and more accurate assessments and recommendations than would be possible using traditional means.

The advantages of clinical decision support systems are numerous:
- **Diagnostic accuracy:** CFs can help to establish a more accurate diagnosis by analysing the patient's symptoms and comparing them with databases of similar cases. This allows for better identification of rare or complex diseases.

- **Treatment optimisation:** By analysing medical data, CFs can recommend specific treatments that are more likely to be successful for a given patient, taking into account their individual characteristics and medical history.

- **Reducing medical errors:** CFs can detect inconsistencies in medical information and recommendations, helping to prevent potentially dangerous errors.

- **Access to up-to-date medical knowledge:** SADCs are regularly updated with the latest medical discoveries and best practices, giving healthcare professionals access to the most up-to-date information for informed decision-making.

- **Improving the efficiency of care:** By providing relevant information and guiding healthcare professionals through the decision-making process, CFDCs can speed up diagnosis and treatment times, thereby improving the efficiency of care.

- **Rationalisation of resources:** CFDCs can help optimise the use of medical resources by identifying the most appropriate treatments and avoiding unnecessary or ineffective treatments.

However, it is essential to note that clinical decision support systems should not be used as substitutes for healthcare professionals. Rather, they should be seen as complementary tools that provide additional information to help clinicians in their decision-making process.

The successful integration of ADAS into clinical practice requires adequate training of healthcare professionals so that they understand how the systems work and know how to interpret the results. In addition, ethical considerations must be taken into account, particularly with regard to the confidentiality of patient data and liability in the event of AI errors.

In conclusion, clinical decision support systems represent a major advance in healthcare, providing valuable information to improve clinical decision-making, optimise treatments and reduce medical errors. With responsible and ethical use, these systems can help to improve the quality of care and patient outcomes.

Anticipating epidemics and outbreaks

Anticipating epidemics and outbreaks is another promising area of application for artificial intelligence (AI) in healthcare. Through the use of AI and massive data analysis, infectious disease outbreaks can be monitored, detected and predicted faster and more accurately than ever before.

Traditionally, epidemic surveillance relied on public health systems that collected data from clinics, laboratories and hospitals, but these methods could be slow and did not always cover large geographical areas. AI, on the other hand, makes it possible to quickly collect, analyse and correlate large amounts of data in real time from multiple sources, such as geographical data, social media, online searches, mobility data and electronic medical records.

Here are some of the ways AI is helping to anticipate epidemics and outbreaks:

- **Early detection:** Machine learning algorithms can analyse data in real time to detect early signs of an outbreak, such as an increase in cases of specific diseases or unusual symptoms reported by patients.

- **Trend forecasting:** AI can analyse historical data from past epidemics to identify trends and patterns of spread, making it possible to predict the geographical areas likely to be affected by a future epidemic.

- **Geographical surveillance:** AI can monitor the movements of populations in real time using location and mobility data, helping to track the spread of diseases and predict their spread to other regions.

- **Social media analysis:** Publications on social networks can provide information about symptoms, local epidemics and risk behaviour. AI can analyse this data to detect early warning signals.

- **Spread modelling:** AI can be used to build models of disease spread, taking into account factors such as transmission rates, virus characteristics and environmental factors.

Using AI to anticipate epidemics and outbreaks enables health authorities to take preventive measures more quickly, such as isolating infected people, monitoring contacts, distributing vaccines and providing early warnings to at-risk populations. These rapid interventions can help to reduce the spread of disease and mitigate the impact of epidemics on public health.

However, it is important to recognise that AI is not infallible and that there are challenges in using these technologies. For example, there can be biases in the algorithms' training data, which can lead to inaccurate predictions or false alerts. In addition, patient confidentiality and privacy must be taken into account when collecting and using health data.

In conclusion, AI plays a key role in anticipating epidemics and outbreaks by enabling real-time surveillance and rapid analysis of health data. Thanks to AI, health authorities can take more effective preventive measures to contain the spread of infectious diseases and protect public health. However, it is important to responsibly manage the challenges associated with the use of AI in epidemiological surveillance, ensuring that the public health benefits are balanced with ethical and data privacy concerns.

The challenge of ethics and confidentiality

The development and use of artificial intelligence (AI) in healthcare raises ethical issues and data privacy challenges. While AI offers many opportunities to improve healthcare, it is essential to consider the ethical implications to ensure responsible and respectful use of sensitive medical data.

Here are some of the key ethical and privacy challenges associated with the use of AI in healthcare:

- **Data privacy:** One of the most significant concerns associated with the use of AI in healthcare is the confidentiality of patient data. AI systems often require sensitive medical data, such as medical records, medical images and genetic test results. It is crucial to ensure that this data is stored, transferred and processed securely to avoid any unauthorised access or breach of privacy.

- **Informed   consent:** The use of medical data for AI raises questions about patients' informed consent. Patients need to be informed in a clear and understandable way about how their data will be used for AI, and they should have the opportunity to give informed consent to participate in these initiatives.

- **Algorithmic biases:** AI algorithms can be subject to biases, as they are based on historical data that may reflect existing inequalities or prejudices in healthcare. This can lead to unfair decisions or differential treatment recommendations for certain groups of patients. It is essential to ensure that algorithms are designed to avoid any potential bias and to be fair to all patients.

- **Transparency and explainability:** Complex AI systems can be difficult to understand and explain, which can cause problems for healthcare professionals and patients. To gain the trust of users, it is crucial that AI systems are transparent and that the decisions they make are explained in a clear and understandable way.

- **Responsibility and accountability:** AI cannot be held responsible for its decisions; responsibility always lies with the designers and users of the systems. It is therefore essential that accountability mechanisms are put in place to ensure that AI is used ethically and in line with best medical practice.

- **Uncertainty and risks:** AI can help in medical decision-making, but it cannot replace the expertise and clinical judgement of healthcare professionals. Errors or misinterpretations of AI results can have serious consequences for patients. It is therefore important to recognise the limitations of AI and put mechanisms in place to mitigate potential risks.

In conclusion, AI offers great opportunities to improve healthcare, but it also poses significant ethical and confidentiality challenges. It is essential to ensure that medical data is used responsibly, ethically and securely, and that decisions made by AI are transparent and explainable. By addressing these ethical issues and ensuring the responsible use of AI, we can take full advantage of this technology to improve healthcare while protecting patient confidentiality and dignity.

Limits and considerations of predictive AI

Predictive AI offers many exciting opportunities to improve healthcare, but it also has important limitations and considerations that need to be taken into account when using it in the medical field. Here are some of the key limitations and considerations of predictive AI:

- **Data quality:** The effectiveness of predictive AI depends largely on the quality of the data used to train the algorithms. If the data is incomplete, inaccurate or biased, AI predictions can be compromised. It is therefore essential to ensure that the medical data used is reliable, complete and representative of the population concerned.

- **Limitations of predictions:** While predictive AI can provide likely estimates of disease risks or medical outcomes, it cannot predict the future with certainty. AI predictions are based on probabilities and historical trends, which means there is always a margin of uncertainty. Clinicians should therefore take these predictions as additional tools to aid decision-making, rather than as definitive results.

- **Problem of overdiagnosis and overtreatment:** The use of predictive AI to detect disease risks can lead to a problem of overdiagnosis, i.e. the diagnosis of diseases that might never have manifested clinically. This can lead to unnecessary or inappropriate treatment, putting patients' health at risk. It is essential to strike a balance between early detection of disease and the risk of over-treatment.

- **Algorithmic bias:** Predictive AI algorithms can be biased depending on the data they are trained on. If the data used to train the AI is biased, this can lead to unfair or discriminatory predictions for certain groups of patients. It is therefore essential to monitor and correct potential biases in algorithms to ensure fairness of predictions.

- **Cost and accessibility:** The implementation of predictive AI systems can be costly, which can limit its access to less financially endowed healthcare establishments. For predictive AI to be widely adopted, costs need to be reduced and it needs to be made accessible to healthcare establishments of all sizes.

- **Privacy and data security:** The use of predictive AI involves the collection and processing of large amounts of sensitive medical data. It is essential to ensure that this data is protected and secured against any unauthorised access or violation of patient privacy.

In conclusion, although predictive AI offers many opportunities to improve healthcare, it also has important limitations and considerations. It is essential to take these factors into account when using predictive AI in clinical practice, ensuring that the data used is of high quality, that predictions are interpreted with caution and that steps are taken to ensure the fairness, confidentiality and security of patient data. With a responsible and ethical approach, predictive AI can be a powerful tool for improving healthcare and patient outcomes.

The future of predictive medicine

The future of predictive medicine is extremely bright, and artificial intelligence (AI) will play an increasingly vital role in this development. As the technology continues to advance, we can expect predictive medicine to become an integral part of healthcare, offering significant benefits to both patients and healthcare professionals.

Here are some of the future prospects for predictive medicine:

- **Prevention and personalised medicine:** Predictive AI will enable more precise identification of individuals at risk of developing certain diseases, opening up opportunities for targeted, personalised prevention. Patients will be able to benefit from lifestyle recommendations and specific treatments based on their genetic profile and individual risk.

- **Early detection of disease:** AI will make it possible to detect early signs of disease even before clinical symptoms appear. This will enable rapid and early intervention, improving the chances of recovery and reducing long-term complications.

- **Personalised treatment:** AI will make it possible to predict a patient's individual response to a given treatment, taking into account their genetic and physiological characteristics. This will lead to more personalised medicine, with treatments tailored to the specific needs of each patient.

- **Improved outcomes for chronic patients:** Patients suffering from chronic diseases will also benefit from predictive AI, which will enable them to monitor changes in their state of health in real time and adjust treatments as their condition fluctuates.

- **Public health surveillance:** Predictive AI will play a crucial role in monitoring epidemics and infectious diseases. It will make it possible to predict epidemic outbreaks, identify disease outbreaks and take preventive measures to contain the spread.

- **Integrating AI into healthcare:** Predictive AI will be integrated into healthcare systems to support healthcare professionals in their clinical decision-making. It will provide real-time recommendations and information to help doctors make informed decisions.

- **Development of new therapies:** Predictive AI will also facilitate the search for new therapies and drugs by identifying potential molecular targets and predicting the efficacy of new treatments.

- **Collaboration between humans and AI:** The future of predictive medicine will not involve replacing healthcare professionals with machines, but rather enabling effective collaboration between the two. Doctors and nurses will use AI as a powerful tool to improve their diagnostic and treatment capabilities.

However, for the future of predictive medicine to be fully realised, challenges will need to be addressed. Data confidentiality, ethical concerns and liability issues will need to be addressed responsibly. In addition, adequate training of healthcare professionals will be essential to ensure effective and ethical use of predictive AI.

In conclusion, predictive AI promises to revolutionise medicine by enabling targeted prevention, early detection of disease and personalised treatment. As a powerful tool for healthcare professionals, predictive AI opens up exciting new opportunities to improve healthcare and patient outcomes. With a responsible and ethical approach, the future of predictive medicine can transform the way we approach health and disease, putting the patient at the centre of healthcare.

Prevention and health promotion

- Artificial intelligence (AI) is playing an increasingly important role in prevention and health promotion. Using sophisticated algorithms and massive data analysis, AI can help identify risk factors, anticipate potential health problems and propose targeted preventive interventions. Here's how AI contributes to prevention and health promotion:

- **Identifying risk factors:** AI can analyse large amounts of health data from a variety of sources, such as electronic medical records, test results, lifestyle habits and genetic data. Using this information, AI can identify individual and population risk factors that contribute to the development of chronic diseases such as diabetes, cardiovascular disease and cancer.

- **Predicting health problems:** Thanks to machine learning and predictive analysis, AI can predict an individual's future health problems based on their medical history and genetic profile. This enables early detection of diseases, facilitating early intervention and the adoption of appropriate preventive measures.

- **Promoting well-being:** AI can also be used to encourage healthy behaviours and promote general wellbeing. AI-enabled health apps can send personalised reminders to patients to help them maintain a balanced diet, exercise regularly and take their medication on time.

- **Personalised treatment:** One of AI's strengths lies in its ability to personalise interventions based on the individual characteristics of each patient. AI can analyse health data to propose prevention programmes tailored to each person's specific needs, optimising the effectiveness of interventions.

- **Public health surveillance:** AI can play a key role in public health surveillance by analysing epidemiological data in real time. This means that epidemics of infectious diseases can be detected quickly and preventive measures put in place to contain their spread.

- **Prediction of complications:** For patients with chronic conditions, AI can predict potential complications based on changes in their health status. This enables healthcare professionals to intervene quickly to avoid serious and costly complications.

- **Reduced healthcare costs:** By anticipating potential health problems and encouraging prevention, AI can help reduce healthcare costs in the long term. Preventing chronic diseases and detecting health problems early can reduce the need for intensive care and costly treatments.

However, it is important to recognise that AI in healthcare is not without its challenges. Data privacy and the security of medical information are major concerns, and it is essential to ensure that patient data is handled ethically and securely. Furthermore, AI should not replace the relationship between patient and healthcare professional, but rather complement it by providing additional information to support decision-making.

In conclusion, AI offers numerous possibilities for improving prevention and health promotion. Thanks to its potential for analysing data and personalising interventions, AI can play a key role in the early detection of disease, the prediction of health risks and the promotion of healthy lifestyles. However, it is essential to consider ethical and confidentiality issues to ensure responsible and respectful use of AI in healthcare. With an ethical and enlightened approach, AI can be a powerful asset for improving the health and well-being of the population.

The nursing robot revolution: How intelligent robots are transforming healthcare

Introduction to intelligent nursing robots

Intelligent nursing robots, also known as care robots or medical assistance robots, represent a major advance in healthcare. These machines with artificial intelligence are designed to interact with patients, provide assistance to healthcare professionals and perform certain medical tasks. Their development has been driven by the need to meet the challenges of an ageing population, a shortage of healthcare staff and growing demand for high-quality healthcare.

Intelligent nursing robots are designed to perform different tasks depending on their capabilities and design. Here are some of their key features and functions:

- **Personal care assistance:** Some nursing robots are designed to help patients with their daily activities, such as getting up, moving around, washing or dressing. They can be equipped with articulated arms, cameras and sensors to interact safely and appropriately with patients.

- **Drug dispensing:** Nursing robots can be programmed to dispense medicines to patients at specific times, ensuring correct dosages and minimising dispensing errors.

- **Monitoring vital signs:** Some robots can be fitted with sensors to monitor patients' vital signs, such as blood pressure, heart rate and temperature, and alert care staff to any worrying variations.

- **Social interaction:** Some nursing robots are designed to interact with patients on a social level, keeping them company, engaging them in conversation or providing them with useful information about their health.

- **Rehabilitation and therapy:** Some robots can be used to help patients recover from injury or surgery by guiding them through rehabilitation or therapy exercises.
- **Delivery of medical supplies:** Nursing robots can also be used to transport medical supplies from one area to another within a healthcare facility, reducing the workload of healthcare professionals.

- **Staff training:** Some robots are used to simulate medical scenarios and train healthcare professionals to react effectively in emergency or complex situations.

However, despite their advantages, intelligent nursing robots also raise important ethical and practical issues. The trust of patients and healthcare professionals in these machines must be established, and it is essential to guarantee the security and confidentiality of the medical data collected by these robots. In addition, it is important to stress that nursing robots cannot completely replace human carers, but rather complement them in certain tasks and provide additional support.

In conclusion, intelligent nursing robots represent an exciting innovation in healthcare. Thanks to their artificial intelligence and versatility, they offer numerous possibilities for improving patient care, relieving the workload of healthcare professionals and optimising the efficiency of healthcare establishments. However, they must be deployed responsibly, taking ethical considerations into account and ensuring that they are used in a way that complements and harmonises with human carers.

Automated nursing robot tasks

Intelligent nursing robots are designed to automate certain tasks in healthcare, which can bring many benefits to patients and medical staff. Here is an overview of the tasks that these robots can perform in an automated way:

- **Assistance with daily activities:** Nursing robots can help patients with their daily activities, such as getting out of bed, sitting up, moving around, washing, brushing their teeth and dressing. They are equipped with articulated arms, cameras and sensors to perform these tasks safely and gently.

- **Dispensing medicines:** Dispensing medication can be a tedious and time-consuming task for care staff. Nursing robots can be programmed to dispense medication to patients at specific times, ensuring correct dosages and reducing the risk of medication errors.

- **Monitoring vital signs:** Some nursing robots are equipped with sensors to monitor patients' vital signs, such as blood pressure, heart rate, oxygen saturation and temperature. They can provide real-time data to nursing staff and alert them to any abnormal values.

- **Collecting and analysing medical data:** Nursing robots can collect and analyse medical data from various sensors and medical devices. They can gather information on a patient's state of health and transmit it to healthcare professionals for informed decision-making.

• **Communication with patients:** Some nursing robots are equipped with voice recognition and text-to-speech functions, enabling them to interact with patients in a friendly and compassionate way. They can answer questions, provide information about treatments and even simply keep patients company.

• **Training and assistance for healthcare professionals:** Nursing robots can be used to simulate medical scenarios and provide practical training for medical students and healthcare professionals. They can also provide assistance in the operating theatre or during medical procedures.

• **Transporting medical supplies:** Some nursing robots are designed to transport medical supplies from one place to another within a healthcare facility. This optimises care logistics and frees up nursing staff for more complex tasks.

It is important to stress that intelligent nursing robots do not replace human carers, but assist them in carrying out certain tasks, allowing them to concentrate on more complex and relational aspects of patient care. Automating these repetitive and time-consuming tasks saves time, reduces errors and optimises the overall efficiency of healthcare.

However, it is essential to ensure that nursing robots are used responsibly and ethically. Patient safety, confidentiality of medical data and transparent communication with patients are key to ensuring the successful and beneficial use of this technology in healthcare.

Assistance for healthcare professionals

Assisting healthcare professionals is one of the main roles of intelligent nursing robots. These machines are designed to work in collaboration with medical staff, supporting them in their daily tasks and improving the overall efficiency of healthcare. Here's how nursing robots can assist healthcare professionals:

- **Handling repetitive tasks:** Nursing robots can perform repetitive and time-consuming tasks, such as dispensing medication, collecting vital data and transporting medical supplies. This allows healthcare professionals to concentrate on more complex and relational tasks.

- **Patient monitoring and follow-up:** Some nursing robots are equipped with sensors to continuously monitor patients' vital signs, movement and activity. This data is then transmitted to healthcare professionals, enabling them to monitor patients' state of health remotely and detect any anomalies quickly.

- **Operating room assistance:** Some nursing robots can be used in the operating room to assist surgeons by providing instruments and supplies, suctioning fluids, maintaining a sterile environment and performing other robot-assisted tasks.

- **Training and simulation:** Nursing robots can be used to simulate medical scenarios, enabling medical students and healthcare professionals to practise complex procedures and interventions in a risk-free environment.

- **Emotional support for patients:** Some nursing robots are designed to interact with patients in a friendly and empathetic way. They can provide a comforting presence to patients and distract them during painful or anxious procedures.

- **Optimised care logistics:** nursing robots can transport medical supplies from one place to another within a healthcare facility, optimising care logistics and reducing waiting times.

- **Reducing the risk of infection:** Nursing robots can be used to perform certain tasks that could otherwise be carried out by healthcare professionals, thereby reducing the risk of nosocomial infection and improving patient safety.

In general, the assistance of nursing robots frees medical staff from repetitive and time-consuming tasks, allowing them to devote more time and attention to patients, treatments and the relational aspects of healthcare. This can improve patient satisfaction, reduce medical errors and improve the overall efficiency of healthcare.

However, it is important to stress that the use of nursing robots does not replace the role of healthcare professionals. They complement the work of human carers and cannot replace the compassion, empathy and human decision-making that are essential in the delivery of quality healthcare. Harmonious collaboration between nursing robots and healthcare professionals is essential to ensure the successful and beneficial use of this technology in healthcare.

Improved efficiency and precision

The introduction of intelligent nursing robots in healthcare establishments has considerably improved the efficiency and accuracy of healthcare. Here's how these machines are contributing to these improvements:

- **Perform repetitive, time-consuming tasks:** Nursing robots are designed to perform repetitive tasks consistently and without fatigue, freeing up time for medical staff to concentrate on more complex, higher added-value tasks.

- **Error-free dispensing of medicines:** Incorrect administration of medicines can have serious consequences for patients. Robotic nurses are programmed to dispense medicines to patients precisely, in the right doses and at the right times, significantly reducing the risk of medication-related medical errors.

- **Continuous patient monitoring:** Some nursing robots are equipped with sensors that enable them to continuously monitor patients' vital signs. They can rapidly detect any abnormal change in a patient's state of health, enabling early intervention and potentially saving lives.

- **Rapid access to medical information:** Robotic nurses can instantly access patients' electronic medical records, test results and drug information, enabling them to provide accurate information to patients and make informed decisions in real time.

- **Precision in medical procedures:** Some nursing robots are used to assist surgeons during medical procedures. Thanks to their stability and precision, these robots can improve the accuracy of surgical gestures and reduce the risk of error.

• **Training healthcare professionals:** Nursing robots can be used as simulators to train medical students and healthcare professionals in complex procedures and situations, enabling them to hone their skills without risk to patients.

• **Optimised care logistics:** nursing robots can transport medical supplies, laboratory samples and other equipment from one place to another quickly and efficiently, saving time and optimising care logistics.

In summary, the use of intelligent nursing robots in healthcare has led to a significant improvement in the efficiency and accuracy of care. These machines automate repetitive tasks, reduce medical errors, continuously monitor patients and provide rapid access to medical information. The result is better quality of care, more positive patient outcomes and more efficient use of medical resources.

However, despite these benefits, it is essential to maintain close oversight of the use of AI in healthcare to ensure responsible and ethical use of these technologies. The trust of patients and medical staff is crucial, and it is important to recognise that nursing robots do not replace human interaction and the expertise of healthcare professionals, but complement them to improve the efficiency of healthcare.

Patient safety and reducing errors

Patient safety is a major concern in healthcare, and the introduction of intelligent nursing robots has the potential to significantly reduce medical errors and improve overall patient safety. Here's how these robots are helping to ensure patient safety:

- **Accurate drug distribution:** Medication errors are one of the main causes of adverse effects in patients. Robotic nurses are programmed to dispense medicines with great precision, following prescribed doses and specific schedules, which considerably reduces the risk of medication-related errors.

- **Continuous monitoring of vital signs:** Some nursing robots are equipped with sensors that enable them to continuously monitor patients' vital signs, such as blood pressure, heart rate and oxygen saturation. By rapidly detecting abnormal variations, these robots can alert medical staff and enable early intervention in the event of a health problem.

- **Prevention of nosocomial infections:** Nursing robots can be used to perform certain tasks that might otherwise be carried out by healthcare professionals, thereby reducing the risk of spreading nosocomial infections. These robots can maintain a sterile environment and avoid cross-contamination.

- **Precision in medical procedures:** Some nursing robots are used to assist surgeons in medical procedures. Thanks to their stability and precision, they can reduce human error and improve the accuracy of surgical gestures.

- **Rapid access to medical information:** Robotic nurses can instantly access patients' electronic medical records and information on prescribed treatments, ensuring that medical staff have all the information they need to make informed decisions and avoid errors.

- **Safe training for healthcare professionals:** Nursing robots can be used as simulators to train medical students and healthcare professionals in complex procedures and situations, enabling them to hone their skills without risk to patients.
- **Reducing manual tasks:** By automating certain tasks, nursing robots reduce reliance on manual tasks performed by healthcare professionals, which can reduce the risk of errors linked to fatigue and burnout.

It is essential to stress that although intelligent nursing robots can improve patient safety, they do not replace the expertise and clinical judgement of healthcare professionals. Robots are designed to assist medical staff in their tasks, but the ultimate responsibility for medical decision-making remains with human carers.

In conclusion, the use of intelligent nursing robots in healthcare has a positive impact on patient safety by reducing medical errors, continuously monitoring vital signs, preventing nosocomial infections and providing rapid access to medical information. By promoting the responsible and ethical use of these technologies, it is possible to further improve patient safety and ensure safe, high-quality care for all.

Communication with patients

Communication with patients is an essential aspect of healthcare, helping to build trust, understand patients' needs and concerns, and provide emotional support. Intelligent nursing robots are designed to interact with patients in a friendly and empathetic way, enhancing the overall healthcare experience. Here's how these robots can facilitate communication with patients:

- **Interactive dialogue:** Some nursing robots are equipped with advanced voice recognition and text-to-speech capabilities, enabling them to engage in interactive dialogue with patients. They can ask questions, answer patients' questions and engage in conversations on various health topics.

- **Answers to frequently asked questions:** The nursing robots can provide answers to questions frequently asked by patients, such as post-operative instructions, side effects of medication, and advice on leading a healthy lifestyle.

- **Treatment information:** Robotic nurses can explain different medical treatments and procedures to patients, providing clear and understandable information about their care plan.

- **Medication and appointment reminders:** Robotic nurses can send reminders to patients to take their medication on time, keep track of their medical appointments and carry out other important tasks related to their treatment.

- **Emotional support:** Some nursing robots are designed to offer emotional support to patients, keeping them company, listening to their concerns and providing comfort at difficult times.

- **Language and cultural adaptation:** Nursing robots can be programmed to communicate in different languages and adapt to different cultures, making it easier to communicate with patients from different backgrounds.

- **Gathering patient feedback:** Nursing robots can collect feedback from patients about their care experience, which can help healthcare facilities improve the quality of the services they offer.

It is important to note that although nursing robots can facilitate communication with patients, they do not replace the human interaction and empathy of healthcare professionals. Human presence remains essential to establish an emotional connection with patients, to detect non-verbal signs and to provide deeper emotional support in complex situations.

Integrating nursing robots into patient communication can be beneficial, particularly in situations where healthcare professionals are overworked or where there are staff shortages. These robots can ease the workload, freeing up time for human carers to concentrate on more complex and relational aspects of healthcare. However, it is essential to ensure that these technologies are used responsibly and ethically, taking into account the confidentiality of patient data and ensuring that communication remains respectful and appropriate.

Integrating robots into healthcare establishments

Integrating intelligent nursing robots into healthcare facilities is a complex process that requires careful planning and close collaboration between healthcare professionals, administrative managers and robot designers. Here are the key steps and considerations for successful integration:

- **Needs assessment:** Before introducing nursing robots into a healthcare facility, it is essential to understand the specific needs of the facility. This involves determining which tasks could be automated, what safety or efficiency issues could be resolved through the use of robots, and how these machines could improve the overall patient experience.

- **Staff training:** The introduction of nursing robots requires adequate training for medical and nursing staff. Staff need to be familiar with how the robots work, how to programme them, monitor them and maintain them properly. They also need to know how to work with the robots to maximise their effectiveness.

- **Selecting the right equipment:** There are different types of nursing robots, each with specific capabilities and functionalities. It is important to choose the equipment that best meets the needs of the healthcare establishment and integrates seamlessly with existing processes and systems.

- **Robot customisation:** Nursing robots can be customised to meet the specific needs of the healthcare organisation and its patients. This can include programming specific questions and answers, adding additional languages to communicate with multilingual patients, and adapting appearances to create a more user-friendly experience.

- **Pilot test:** Before deploying robots on a large scale, it is advisable to carry out a pilot test in a limited area of the facility. This allows you to gather feedback from staff and patients, identify any problems and fine-tune the process before full implementation.

- **Patient and data safety:** Patient safety and the confidentiality of medical data are paramount when integrating robots into healthcare. Robots must be equipped with robust security measures to protect sensitive patient information and avoid any risk of cyber attacks.

- **Communication and acceptance:** Transparent communication with patients, families and staff is essential to explain the benefits of introducing nursing robots and to allay any concerns about the use of technology in healthcare.

- **Ongoing monitoring:** Once the robots have been deployed, it is important to monitor their operation and impact on healthcare on an ongoing basis. This allows any problems to be detected quickly and improvements implemented if necessary.

In summary, the integration of intelligent nursing robots into healthcare facilities offers many opportunities to improve the efficiency, accuracy and safety of care. However, careful planning, adequate training and transparent communication are essential for the successful and beneficial implementation of this technology. Nursing robots do not replace human carers, but they can be valuable assistants in improving patient experience and optimising care processes.

Acceptance by healthcare professionals and patients

The acceptance of nursing robots by healthcare professionals and patients is an essential aspect of their successful integration into healthcare establishments. Here are some key points concerning the acceptance of this technology by these two groups:

Acceptance by healthcare professionals :
- **Adequate training:** Healthcare professionals must be properly trained in the use of nursing robots, their capabilities and their limitations. Comprehensive training helps to dispel concerns and build confidence in this technology.

- **Understanding the benefits:** The benefits of nursing robots need to be clearly explained to healthcare professionals. It is essential to highlight how these machines can relieve repetitive tasks, improve the accuracy of care and allow carers to concentrate on more complex and relational tasks.

- **Involvement in the decision:** Involving healthcare professionals in the decision to integrate nursing robots into their practice fosters a sense of control and commitment to this technology.

- **Ongoing communication:** Open and ongoing communication between robot designers and healthcare professionals is essential to resolve any problems or concerns quickly and to adapt robots to real needs.

- **Opportunities for improvement:** Encouraging healthcare professionals to provide feedback on the use of robots and suggest improvements can contribute to the acceptance and adoption of this technology.

Patient acceptance :

- **Information and education:** Patients need to be informed about the use of nursing robots and their role in healthcare. Appropriate education can help to dispel fears and create a clear understanding of the benefits of these robots.

- **User-friendly experience:** Nursing robots must be designed to be user-friendly and reassuring for patients. Their appearance, voice and behaviour must be adapted to facilitate positive interaction.

- **Access to care:** If nursing robots can help improve access to care and reduce waiting times, this may be a deciding factor for patients in favour of this technology.

- **Respect for privacy and confidentiality:** Patients must be assured that nursing robots respect their privacy and that their medical information is secure.

- **Patient satisfaction:** Once the nursing robots have been deployed, measuring patient satisfaction with their use can help to assess their acceptance and identify potential areas for improvement.

In short, the acceptance of nursing robots by healthcare professionals and patients is a complex process that requires a considered approach. By providing adequate training, communicating transparently and focusing on the benefits to healthcare, successful adoption of this technology can be fostered. While recognising that nursing robots do not replace human interaction, they can be valuable tools for improving healthcare and enhancing efficiency, safety and the overall patient experience.

The complementary role of robot nurses

Nursing robots play an essential complementary role in healthcare establishments, where they assist human healthcare professionals to improve the quality of care and optimise work processes. Here's how these robots play a complementary role in healthcare:

- **Automating repetitive tasks:** Robotic nurses can take on repetitive and time-consuming tasks, such as dispensing medicines at set times, collecting biological samples and monitoring vital signs. This frees up time for healthcare professionals, who can then concentrate on more complex tasks requiring their human expertise and sensitivity.
- **Accuracy and error reduction:** Nursing robots are programmed to perform tasks with great accuracy, significantly reducing the risk of human error. They can also rigorously follow care protocols and adhere to prescribed doses and schedules, improving patient safety.
- **Continuous patient monitoring:** Some nursing robots are equipped with sensors that enable them to constantly monitor patients' vital signs. By rapidly detecting any abnormal changes, these robots can alert medical staff for early intervention in the event of complications.
- **Rapid access to medical information:** Robotic nurses can instantly access patients' electronic medical records, test results and information on prescribed treatments. This means they can provide

accurate, up-to-date information to patients and medical staff.

- **Emotional support:** Some nursing robots are designed to offer emotional support to patients, providing comfort and companionship. Although they cannot replace human empathy, their presence can help to alleviate loneliness and anxiety in some patients.

- **Training and learning:** Nursing robots can be used as simulators to train medical students and healthcare professionals in complex procedures and situations. In this way, they offer a safe and risk-free learning opportunity for future carers.

- **Optimising resources:** The use of nursing robots makes it possible to optimise human and material resources in healthcare establishments. They can help reduce staff workloads, improve care efficiency and optimise care logistics.

-

It is important to emphasise that nursing robots do not replace human healthcare professionals. On the contrary, they complement them to improve the quality of care, facilitate the work of medical staff and enhance the patient experience. Healthcare remains a discipline in which empathy, communication and taking into account the emotional dimension of patients play an essential role, and these aspects can only be fully handled by human carers. The interaction between nursing robots and human healthcare professionals offers a unique potential for synergy to create a more efficient and humane care environment.

Ethics of Autonomy:
The Dilemmas of AI in Clinical Decision Making

Introduction to AI-based decision support systems

Artificial intelligence (AI)-based decision support systems are powerful tools that combine medical expertise with the advanced analytical capabilities of AI to help healthcare professionals make informed and accurate decisions. These systems are designed to provide information and recommendations based on medical data and scientific evidence to help clinicians diagnose, plan treatments and manage care more effectively. Here's how AI-based decision support systems work:

- **Data collection and analysis:** Decision support systems collect and analyse large amounts of medical data from a variety of sources, such as electronic medical records, test results, medical images and genetic data. AI uses sophisticated algorithms to extract relevant information and identify patterns hidden in this data.

- **Diagnosis and prediction:** Thanks to data analysis, decision support systems can help doctors to make more accurate and faster diagnoses. They can also help predict the risk of certain diseases in patients by analysing their individual characteristics and medical history.

- **Treatment recommendations :** Decision support systems can recommend appropriate treatments based on the patient's diagnosis and available clinical evidence. These recommendations can be personalised according to the patient's individual characteristics, such as genetic profile and treatment preferences.

- **Healthcare management:** These systems can also help clinicians to plan and manage care more effectively by optimising available resources, following treatment protocols and monitoring patient outcomes.

- **Continuing education:** Decision support systems can be used as continuing education tools for healthcare professionals. By analysing clinical cases and proposing learning scenarios, these systems can improve clinicians' skills and keep them abreast of the latest medical advances.

- **Prevention and public health:** These systems can play a crucial role in disease prevention by identifying risk factors in individuals and proposing preventive interventions. They can also contribute to public health by detecting emerging epidemics and recommending intervention measures.

- **Improved decision-making:** By providing evidence-based information, decision support systems help clinicians to make more informed decisions and avoid the cognitive biases that can influence human judgements.

It is important to note that while AI-based decision support systems offer many benefits, they should never replace the clinical judgement of healthcare professionals. These systems should be seen as assistive tools that support medical decisions, but ultimately it is clinicians who are responsible for patient care. Trust and understanding of these systems by healthcare professionals is essential to ensure effective and responsible use of AI in healthcare.

Transparency and interpretability of algorithms

The transparency and interpretability of artificial intelligence (AI) algorithms are crucial to gaining the trust of healthcare professionals and patients in the use of these technologies. When it comes to making important medical decisions, it is essential to understand how AI arrives at its conclusions and the basis on which it makes its recommendations. Here's why the transparency and interpretability of algorithms is so important in healthcare:

- **Clinician confidence:** Healthcare professionals need to be able to trust the results provided by AI systems. When algorithms are transparent and easy to interpret, clinicians can better understand how decisions are made and are more likely to accept and follow AI recommendations.
- **Informed decision-making:** Transparent AI enables clinicians to make informed decisions and assess the validity of results. The explanations provided by the AI give a better understanding of the underlying reasons for its recommendations, helping clinicians to take all relevant factors into account in their decision-making.

- **Responsibility and accountability:** The transparency of algorithms makes it easier to understand the factors taken into account by AI and to know whether biases or errors can influence the results. This makes algorithm designers more accountable for the quality of their models and the decisions they generate.

- **Patient understanding:** For patients, understanding the reasons why a treatment has been recommended by the AI is essential to encourage adherence to care. The interpretability of algorithms means that the reasons behind medical decisions can be explained more clearly, boosting patient confidence in the care process.

- **Error detection and correction:** When algorithms are transparent, errors or biases can be more easily detected and corrected. This improves the quality and safety of the healthcare provided by AI.

- **Regulatory compliance:** In many countries, there are strict regulations regarding the use of AI in medicine, including data protection and patient confidentiality. Algorithm transparency ensures that AI systems comply with these rules and standards.

However, it is important to note that some types of AI algorithms, such as deep neural networks, can be inherently complex and difficult to interpret. Progress is being made to make these models more understandable, but it can be difficult to provide a full explanation of every decision made by the AI.

Transparent and interpretable AI is a major objective of artificial intelligence research. Algorithm designers and researchers are working to develop methods that provide clear explanations of the reasoning behind AI systems, without sacrificing their performance. Ultimately, improving the transparency and interpretability of AI algorithms is essential to ensure responsible and ethical use of this powerful technology in healthcare.

Bias and fairness in AI models

Biases in artificial intelligence (AI) models are a major concern in healthcare. When algorithms are trained on data sets that are unbalanced or contain systemic biases, they can reproduce these biases when making decisions. This can lead to inequalities in healthcare and negatively affect certain groups of patients. Here are some key points about bias and fairness in AI models:

- **Bias in the data:** Biases in AI models often come from the data on which these models are trained. If historical data contains disparities in patient treatment or misdiagnoses, the algorithm risks perpetuating these inequalities. For example, if patients of a certain race or gender were misdiagnosed or undertreated in the past, the AI could reproduce these patterns.

- **Impact on vulnerable groups:** Biases in AI models can have a disproportionate impact on vulnerable groups, such as racial minorities, people on low incomes or marginalised populations. This can lead to unequal access to healthcare, misdiagnosis or inappropriate treatment for these populations.

- **Health equity:** Health equity is an important goal in healthcare, aiming to ensure equal access to care and equitable health outcomes for all individuals, regardless of their social origin, race, gender or economic status. Biases in AI models can hinder this objective by perpetuating existing inequalities.

- **Bias detection and mitigation:** Researchers and algorithm designers are actively working on the detection and mitigation of biases in AI models. Methods such as data balancing, algorithmic bias reduction and the use of fairness metrics are being explored to ensure that AI models are more equitable and respectful of patient diversity.

- **Transparency and accountability:** The transparency of AI models is essential to understanding the factors that influence medical decisions. Algorithm developers must be responsible for detecting and correcting biases in their models to ensure responsible use of AI in healthcare.

- **Ethical training for healthcare professionals:** Healthcare professionals must be made aware of the problems of bias in AI and trained in the responsible use of these technologies. They play a key role in supervising and validating the decisions made by AI, ensuring that recommendations are fair and consistent with the ethical principles of medicine.

Fairness in AI models is a complex challenge that requires a multidisciplinary and collaborative approach. It is essential that algorithm developers, AI researchers, healthcare professionals, policy makers and patients work together to ensure that AI in healthcare is used ethically and responsibly, with a focus on equity, accessibility and quality of care for all.

Responsibility and accountability in AI decisions

Responsibility and accountability are crucial aspects of the use of artificial intelligence (AI) in healthcare. When important medical decisions are made in part or in whole by AI systems, it is essential to establish accountability mechanisms to ensure the quality, safety and ethics of care. Here are some key points about responsibility and accountability in healthcare AI decisions:

- **Responsibility of algorithm designers:** AI algorithm designers are responsible for the quality of the models they develop. They must ensure that the models are properly trained, validated and tested before they are deployed in clinical environments. They must also take into account the potential biases and risks associated with the decisions made by the AI.

- **Transparency of decisions:** The decisions made by AI systems must be transparent and explainable. Algorithm designers must provide mechanisms to explain how AI arrives at its conclusions, so that healthcare professionals and patients can understand the reasons behind these decisions.

- **Human supervision:** Even when AI plays an important role in decision-making, human supervision remains essential. Healthcare professionals must always supervise and validate AI decisions, using their clinical expertise to make informed decisions.

- **Error identification:** Mechanisms must be put in place to detect and correct any errors in AI decisions. This may include regular audits, peer reviews and processes for reporting errors by healthcare professionals.

- **Training and education:** Healthcare professionals need to be trained in the use of AI in healthcare and in understanding its limitations and risks. This also includes awareness of how to work with AI systems to make ethical and informed decisions.

- **Responsibility of healthcare organisations:** Healthcare organisations using AI systems are also responsible for their ethical and responsible use. They must have policies and procedures in place to ensure that AI is used appropriately and in compliance with applicable standards and regulations.

- **Accountability to patients:** Patients have a right to know how medical decisions affecting them are made, whether by healthcare professionals or AI systems. Healthcare organisations must be transparent with patients about the use of AI in care and ensure that patients are informed of their rights and treatment choices.

Accountability and responsibility are key to ensuring the ethical and responsible use of AI in healthcare. By focusing on transparency, human supervision and adequate training of healthcare professionals, it is possible to get the most out of AI while maintaining safety and quality of care for patients.

Autonomy and shared decision-making

The integration of artificial intelligence (AI) into healthcare raises important questions about patient autonomy and shared decision-making between patients and healthcare professionals. Autonomy is the right of patients to make informed decisions about their health, while shared decision-making is a collaborative approach between patient and healthcare professional to develop a treatment plan that takes into account the patient's values and preferences. Here's how AI can influence patient autonomy and shared decision-making:

- **Access to information:** AI gives patients access to a considerable amount of information about their health and treatment options. This strengthens their ability to make informed decisions and play an active role in their own care.

- **Personalised care:** AI can help to personalise care by analysing individual patient data, such as medical history, test results and personal preferences. This allows treatment plans to be tailored to each patient, respecting their autonomy.

- **Transparent explanations:** When AI is used to make medical decisions, it is essential to provide clear and understandable explanations to patients about the reasons behind these decisions. This helps patients understand recommendations and make informed decisions in collaboration with their care team.

- **Limitations of AI:** Although AI is a valuable tool, it does have its limitations. Patients need to be aware that AI does not replace the clinical judgement of healthcare professionals, but it can help them make informed decisions.

- **Privacy:** The use of AI to analyse medical data can raise privacy concerns. Patients need to be assured that their data is protected and used ethically, which can increase their confidence in the use of AI in healthcare.

- **Communication and education:** To facilitate effective shared decision-making, it is essential that healthcare professionals communicate clearly with patients and educate them about the benefits and limitations of AI in healthcare.

- **Consideration of the patient's values:** In shared decision-making, healthcare professionals must take into account the patient's values, beliefs and preferences. AI can provide objective information, but the final decision should always reflect the patient's needs and choices.

Ultimately, the integration of AI into healthcare can empower patients and support more informed shared decision-making. However, it is essential to ensure that the use of AI is ethical, transparent and respectful of patients' rights and preferences. By focusing on education, communication and privacy protection, AI can be used as a powerful tool to improve healthcare decision-making while respecting patient autonomy.

Informed consent for the use of AI

Informed consent is a fundamental principle of medical ethics which ensures that patients fully understand the risks, benefits and implications of their treatment or participation in medical research. When it comes to the use of artificial intelligence (AI) in healthcare, informed consent takes on particular importance due to the complexity of this technology. Here are some points to consider regarding informed consent for the use of AI:

- **Explaining the use of AI:** Patients need to be informed that AI may be used in their medical care, and it is important to explain to them in understandable terms how AI works, what information will be used and how this may influence medical decisions affecting them.

- **Risks and benefits:** Patients should be informed of the potential risks associated with the use of AI, such as data bias or misinterpretation, as well as the benefits, such as faster and more accurate diagnoses or personalised treatment recommendations.

- **Use of data:** The use of AI often involves the analysis of large amounts of patient medical data. Informed consent must include information on how this data will be used, stored and protected to ensure the confidentiality and security of the patient's personal information.

- **Right of refusal:** Patients have the right to refuse the use of AI in their medical care. They must be informed of this possibility and be assured that such a refusal will not have a negative impact on the quality of their care.

- **Understanding and questions:** Informed consent implies that patients fully understand the information provided and have the opportunity to ask questions to clarify any points that may be ambiguous.

- **Consent updates:** The use of AI in healthcare may evolve over time, and patients should be informed of any significant changes in the use of AI and given the opportunity to provide informed consent again.

- **Specific   consent:** In some cases, the use of AI may be specific to a particular medical field or type of treatment. Informed consent must be adapted accordingly to reflect these specificities.

Informed consent for the use of AI is essential to respect patients' rights to self-determination and informed decision-making about their health. Healthcare professionals have a responsibility to ensure that patients fully understand the implications of using AI in their medical care and to respect their choice regarding its use. Fostering clear and transparent communication with patients can promote the responsible and ethical use of AI in healthcare while respecting patients' rights and preferences.

The role of human expertise

Despite the rapid advances in artificial intelligence (AI) in healthcare, human expertise remains irreplaceable and plays an essential role in the delivery of quality healthcare. Here are some key points on the place of human expertise in the context of the use of AI in healthcare:

- **Ethical decision-making:** Human expertise is needed to address the complex ethical issues that can arise in healthcare. Healthcare professionals can factor ethical, social and cultural considerations into their decisions, taking into account patient preferences and considering the long-term implications.

- **Empathy and compassion:** Healthcare is first and foremost a relationship between patient and carer. Human expertise enables us to create empathetic links and provide emotional support to patients, which is essential for improving their psychological and physical well-being.

- **Individual context:** Every patient is unique, with individual needs and characteristics. Human expertise enables us to take these specificities into account and adapt care to suit each individual case.

- **Flexibility and adaptability:** Healthcare professionals can be faced with unforeseen or complex situations that may escape AI algorithms. Their expertise enables them to provide flexible, tailored solutions in unique scenarios.

- **Communication:** Interacting with patients and communicating complex information are crucial human skills in healthcare. The ability to explain

99

medical concepts in an understandable and empathetic way is essential for involving patients in their treatment.

- **Critical evaluation of AI results:** While AI can help provide information and recommendations, healthcare professionals must always be able to critically evaluate these results to ensure their accuracy and clinical relevance.

- **Creativity and problem solving:** Human expertise enables creativity and critical thinking to solve complex problems that may be beyond the capabilities of AI.

The integration of AI into healthcare offers many opportunities to improve diagnosis, treatment and patient outcomes. However, human expertise remains essential to complement the capabilities of AI and ensure high-quality, ethical and patient-centred healthcare. The cohabitation of AI with human expertise will make the most of both worlds, creating a more comprehensive and efficient healthcare system that puts patient wellbeing at its heart.

Limits and uncertainties of AI systems

While artificial intelligence (AI) offers many opportunities and promises in healthcare, there are also limitations and uncertainties associated with its use. Here are some of the main limitations and uncertainties of AI systems in healthcare:

- **Lack of explainability:** AI models, particularly deep neural networks, can be complex and difficult to explain. It can be difficult for healthcare professionals to understand how AI arrives at its conclusions, which can lead to a loss of confidence in its use.

- **Quality data:** AI systems require high-quality data sets to function optimally. If the data is incomplete, unbalanced or contains errors, this can affect the accuracy and reliability of the AI results.

- **Bias in the data:** The data used to train AI models may contain biases and inequalities that can be reproduced by AI. This can lead to unfair treatment recommendations for certain groups of patients.

- **Diagnostic limitations:** While AI can be valuable in helping to diagnose certain conditions, it cannot replace human expertise in all situations. Some diagnoses can be complex and require a comprehensive assessment of the patient by a healthcare professional.

- **Risk of overconfidence:** Overconfidence in AI systems can lead to overdependence on the technology, which can lead to errors if AI results are not properly verified by healthcare professionals.

- **Lack of empathy:** AI lacks emotion and empathy, which can be a limiting factor in interactions with patients, particularly in emotional or sensitive situations.

- **Cybersecurity and data protection:** The use of AI in healthcare involves the collection and use of large amounts of personal patient data. This raises cybersecurity and data protection concerns, as AI systems can be vulnerable to attacks and privacy breaches.

- **Cost and accessibility:** Implementing AI in healthcare establishments can be costly, which may limit access for certain establishments or regions with limited resources.

Despite these limitations and uncertainties, it is important to recognise that AI has the potential to transform healthcare in a positive way. By understanding the limits of AI and working responsibly and ethically, we can reap its benefits while minimising the potential risks. A balanced approach, integrating human expertise and AI in a complementary way, can optimise patient outcomes and improve healthcare as a whole.

Ethical standards for AI systems in healthcare

Artificial intelligence (AI) systems in healthcare must be subject to rigorous ethical standards to ensure that they are used responsibly, fairly and safely. Here are some important ethical standards to consider for AI systems in healthcare:

- **Transparency and explicability:** AI systems must be transparent in their operation and decisions. Algorithm designers must explain how AI arrives at its conclusions so that healthcare professionals and patients can understand the reasons behind these decisions.

- **Fairness and absence of bias:** AI systems must not reproduce existing biases in training data. Steps must be taken to ensure that AI recommendations are fair and do not unduly favour certain groups of patients.

- **Privacy and data protection:** Patient medical data is highly sensitive and must be treated with the utmost respect for privacy. AI systems must be designed to guarantee data confidentiality, security and integrity.

- **Responsibility and accountability:** Developers and users of AI systems in healthcare must be held accountable for their actions. There must be accountability mechanisms in place to detect and correct potential errors and to address complaints related to the use of AI.

- **Shared decision-making:** AI systems in healthcare should be designed to complement and enhance shared decision-making between patients and healthcare professionals, not to replace this collaborative approach.

- **Ethical use of AI:** AI systems in healthcare should be used to improve patient care and well-being, not to harm or exploit individuals.

- **Training and education:** Healthcare professionals and algorithm designers must be trained in the ethical use of AI in healthcare and in understanding its ethical and social implications.

- **Independent evaluation:** AI systems in healthcare need to be independently evaluated to ensure their ethical compliance and safety.

- **Informed consent:** Patients must be informed of the use of AI in their medical care and must give their informed consent for this use.
- **Limits and uncertainties:** The limits and uncertainties of AI systems in healthcare must be clearly communicated to healthcare professionals and patients for informed decision-making.

By following these ethical standards, a responsible and ethical use of AI in healthcare can be promoted, ensuring that this innovative technology truly benefits patients and contributes to improving healthcare in an equitable and sustainable way. It is essential that those involved in the development and use of AI in healthcare work together to promote an ethical culture that puts the well-being of patients first.

Outlook for the future: The evolution of AI in clinical decision-making

The outlook for the future of artificial intelligence (AI) in clinical decision-making is promising and full of possibilities. AI will continue to evolve and develop in healthcare, bringing significant improvements in the way healthcare professionals make clinical decisions. Here are some key prospects for the future:

- **Improved diagnostic accuracy:** AI systems will continue to improve in the early and accurate detection of diseases, enabling faster and more reliable diagnosis. AI can be particularly useful in identifying rare or complex diseases.

- **Personalised treatment:** AI will provide a better understanding of inter-individual variation in response to treatments. By analysing large quantities of medical data, AI will be able to help personalise treatments for each patient based on their unique characteristics.

- **Enhanced shared decision-making:** AI can support healthcare professionals and patients to facilitate more informed shared decision-making. The information provided by AI can help patients better understand their treatment options and associated risks, encouraging their active participation in their own care.

- **Chronic disease management:** AI can be used to monitor patients with chronic diseases in real time and provide personalised management recommendations. This can help improve disease control and avoid complications.

- **Early detection of epidemics:** AI can be used to monitor epidemiological trends on a global scale and detect early warning signals of potential outbreaks. This will enable a faster and more effective response to future epidemics.

- **Improved explanation and interpretability:** Researchers are working on approaches to make AI models more explainable and interpretable. This will enable healthcare professionals to better understand the decisions made by AI and increase their confidence in its use.

- **Seamless integration into care practices:** As AI progresses, it will become more integrated into healthcare systems and the workflows of healthcare professionals. The use of AI will become smoother and more intuitive, allowing clinicians to reap its full benefits.

- **Training and education:** AI will require ongoing training for healthcare professionals to ensure appropriate and ethical use of this technology. Training programmes will be developed to enhance skills in the use of AI in healthcare.

- **Collaboration with industry:** AI will continue to be developed in partnership with the technology industry, opening up new opportunities for innovation and advances in healthcare.

* **Regulatory developments:** As the use of AI in healthcare becomes more widespread, regulations and ethical standards will be updated to ensure responsible and safe use of the technology.

In sum, AI represents a major evolution in clinical decision-making that will continue to reshape healthcare practices for years to come. A focus on ethics, transparency and improved patient care will be key to realising the full potential of AI in healthcare. By collaborating responsibly, healthcare professionals and AI developers can create an integrated future where AI and human expertise come together to deliver high-quality, patient-centric healthcare.

Tracking down epidemics: How AI is helping to prevent global health crises

Introduction to AI-based epidemiological surveillance

The introduction of epidemiological surveillance based on artificial intelligence (AI) marks a significant step forward in the management of global health crises. Epidemiological surveillance is the process of collecting, analysing and continuously interpreting health data to detect and monitor outbreaks of infectious diseases and notifiable diseases. The use of AI in this area brings many benefits, enabling early detection of outbreaks, rapid response and informed decision-making to prevent the spread of disease.

How AI-based epidemiological surveillance works :
- **Real-time data collection:** AI makes it possible to collect data in real time from a variety of sources, such as electronic medical records, disease surveillance systems, social media and health sensors. This data is aggregated and analysed to detect trends and deviations that could indicate an emerging epidemic.

- **Early detection of epidemics:** Using machine learning algorithms, AI can identify anomalies in health data and detect patterns that could indicate the start of an epidemic. This enables health authorities to take swift action to contain the spread before it gets out of control.

- **Monitoring population movements:** AI can track population movements using geolocation and transport data. This helps predict the spread of disease and identify high-risk areas.

- **Massive data analysis:** AI-based epidemiological surveillance can analyse large quantities of data in record time, enabling complex patterns and epidemiological trends to be detected quickly.

- **Epidemic modelling:** AI algorithms can be used to model the spread of epidemics and predict their future evolution. This helps health managers to plan the resources needed to deal with the crisis.

- **Decision-making support:** AI provides factual information and in-depth analyses to help decision-makers make informed decisions about the public health measures to be taken to control the epidemic.

- **Early warning systems:** AI can be integrated into early warning systems that automatically alert health authorities to signs of impending epidemics, enabling a rapid response.

Advantages of AI-based epidemiological surveillance :
- **Speed:** AI can analyse large quantities of data in real time, enabling emerging epidemics to be detected and responded to quickly.

- **Accuracy:** Machine learning algorithms can detect complex patterns and trends in data, improving the accuracy of epidemiological surveillance.

- **Adaptability:** AI can adapt quickly to changes in epidemics and provide health managers with up-to-date information.

- **Effective resource planning:** By modelling the spread of epidemics, AI enables better resource planning and a more effective response.

- **Preventing the spread:** By detecting epidemics at an early stage, AI can help prevent them from spreading on a large scale.

In conclusion, the introduction of AI-based epidemiological surveillance represents a major advance in the management of global health crises. Thanks to its ability to analyse data quickly and accurately, AI plays a key role in the early detection of epidemics, the efficient planning of resources and the prevention of the spread of disease. However, it is important to stress that AI is a complementary tool and does not replace the expertise and judgement of healthcare professionals in managing epidemics.

Real-time data collection and analysis

Real-time data collection and analysis are essential elements of epidemiological surveillance based on artificial intelligence (AI). This approach enables the rapid detection of emerging trends and anomalies in health data, facilitating the early detection of epidemics and rapid decision-making in public health. Here's how real-time data collection and analysis is achieved:

Real-time data collection :
- **Health sensors:** Health sensors, such as wearable devices, medical monitors and remote monitoring

devices, can collect real-time data on patients' vital signs, such as heart rate, blood pressure, temperature and oxygen saturation.

- **Electronic medical records (EMR):** EMRs enable patient medical data to be stored and accessed electronically. This makes information on medical visits, diagnoses, laboratory results and treatments available to healthcare professionals in real time.

- **Social media monitoring:** AI can be used to monitor social media for mentions of disease symptoms or epidemic situations. This can provide clues about potential disease outbreaks.

- **Transport surveillance:** real-time geolocation and transport data can be used to track population movements and identify areas at high risk of epidemics.

- **Environmental data:** Collecting environmental data, such as air pollution levels, weather conditions and water quality data, can help to understand the environmental factors that could influence the spread of disease.

Real-time data analysis :
- **Machine learning algorithms:** AI uses machine learning algorithms to analyse data in real time and detect patterns and trends. These algorithms can identify deviations from norms and warn of potentially problematic situations.

- **Predictive modelling:** AI-based predictive models can be used to anticipate the spread of epidemics. Using current data, these models can predict how the epidemiological situation will evolve over the coming days and weeks.

- **Early warning systems:** AI can be used to develop early warning systems that rapidly detect emerging epidemics and send alerts to health authorities for a rapid response.

- **Identification of epidemic outbreaks:** Real-time data analysis can be used to identify geographical areas where epidemic outbreaks could occur, enabling health officials to focus their prevention and control efforts.

- **Monitoring health behaviours:** Real-time data analysis can be used to monitor the health behaviours of the population, such as use of health services, use of medication and compliance with preventive measures.

In conclusion, the collection and analysis of real-time data using AI play a crucial role in epidemiological surveillance and the management of health crises. These approaches make it possible to detect emerging epidemics quickly, track their spread, plan resources efficiently and make informed public health decisions. The ability to collect and analyse data in real time enables a faster and more accurate response to epidemics, helping to reduce their impact on public health.

Early identification of epidemics

Early identification of epidemics is crucial to preventing their rapid spread and to taking effective public health measures. Thanks to the use of artificial intelligence (AI) and real-time data collection, it is possible to rapidly detect the early warning signals that indicate the start of an epidemic. Here's how AI plays a key role in the early identification of epidemics:

- **Real-time health data monitoring:** AI can rapidly collect, aggregate and analyse real-time health data from a variety of sources, such as electronic medical records, disease surveillance systems, social media, health sensors and epidemiological reports. By analysing this data in real time, AI can detect unusual trends and deviations that could indicate a sudden increase in cases of disease.

- **Detection of emerging patterns and trends:** Using machine learning algorithms, AI can quickly identify patterns and trends that could be characteristic of an emerging epidemic. For example, if a significant increase in cases of similar symptoms is observed in a given region, AI can alert health authorities to the possibility of an epidemic in progress.

- **Analysis of online search behaviour:** AI can monitor individuals' online search behaviour, such as searches for disease symptoms or preventive measures. Significant changes in these behaviours can serve as early indicators of an emerging epidemic.

- **Use of early warning systems:** AI can be integrated into early warning systems that automatically identify early warning signals and send alerts to health officials for immediate action.
- **Geospatial analysis:** AI can use geolocation data to monitor population movements and identify areas where epidemic outbreaks could occur. This enables a rapid, targeted response in these high-risk areas.

- **Comparison with historical data:** AI can analyse historical data on previous epidemics and compare it with current data to detect any significant or unusual changes in epidemiological patterns.

-

By combining the power of AI with real-time data collection, epidemiological surveillance systems can become much more responsive and effective in the early identification of epidemics. This enables health officials to take rapid action to contain the spread of the disease, isolate confirmed cases and implement appropriate prevention measures. Early identification of epidemics plays a key role in preventing major health crises, and AI offers a valuable tool for strengthening this early detection capability and reacting quickly to protect public health.

Predictive modelling of epidemics

Predictive epidemic modelling is a powerful application of artificial intelligence (AI) in the field of public health. This approach uses machine learning algorithms to analyse historical and real-time epidemiological data to predict the future course of an epidemic. Predictive modelling plays a crucial role in public health decision-making, enabling health authorities to plan and implement prevention and control measures in a more informed and proactive way. Here's how predictive modelling of epidemics is achieved using AI:

- **Epidemiological data collection:** Predictive modelling begins with the collection of epidemiological data, such as the number of confirmed cases, the number of deaths, the geolocation of cases, risk factors, rates of spread, and so on. These data can come from a variety of sources, including disease surveillance systems, epidemiological reports, electronic medical records and government databases.

- **Data pre-processing:** Before applying machine learning algorithms, epidemiological data must be pre-processed to eliminate outliers, fill in missing data and normalise the data to ensure the quality and consistency of the data used for analysis.

- **Feature selection:** Epidemiological data can contain numerous variables and features. AI can be used to select the most relevant features for analysis and prediction, improving model accuracy.

- **Predictive models:** Using machine learning algorithms, predictive models are built using historical epidemiological data. These models can be based on various algorithms, such as neural networks, random forests, support vector machines, etc.

- **Model validation:** Predictive models need to be validated using independent data to assess their accuracy and reliability in predicting epidemics.

- **Forecasting the evolution of the epidemic: Once** the predictive models have been validated, they are used to forecast the future evolution of the epidemic. These forecasts can include projections on the number of future cases, geographical spread, duration of the epidemic, etc.

- **Planning public health measures:** The forecasts generated by predictive modelling help health managers to plan and implement appropriate public health measures to control the epidemic. These may include vaccination campaigns, quarantine measures, travel restrictions, etc.

AI makes predictive modelling of epidemics faster, more accurate and more proactive. It enables healthcare managers to make informed decisions to protect public health, prevent the spread of disease and better manage health crises. Predictive modelling is a valuable tool in the toolbox of healthcare professionals to meet the challenges posed by epidemics and help save lives.

Global Public Health Surveillance

Global public health surveillance is a crucial area for detecting, preventing and responding to global health threats such as epidemics, pandemics and emerging infectious diseases. The use of artificial intelligence (AI) in global public health surveillance brings significant benefits by improving large-scale data collection and analysis, early detection of epidemics and international coordination of public health efforts. Here's how AI is playing a key role in global public health surveillance:

- **Large-scale data collection:** AI facilitates the collection, aggregation and analysis of health data from multiple, geographically dispersed sources. This includes disease surveillance systems, electronic medical records, government databases, epidemiological reports, social media and health sensors, among others. This large-scale data collection allows us to better understand global health trends and identify emerging health issues.

- **Early detection of epidemics:** AI is used to analyse epidemiological data in real time and detect early warning signs of an emerging epidemic. AI-based predictive models can identify abnormal trends and unusual patterns in the data, enabling early detection of potential epidemics.

- **International travel monitoring:** AI can monitor large-scale international travel, such as air travel, to identify risks of rapid disease spread between countries. This enables health officials to take preventive measures to limit the cross-border spread of disease.

- **Geospatial analysis:** AI uses geolocation data to map the spread of diseases, identify high-risk areas and assess the effectiveness of control measures put in place.

- **Social media monitoring:** AI is used to monitor social media and online platforms to quickly detect mentions of disease symptoms, red flags and potential rumours about public health issues.

- **International collaboration:** AI facilitates collaboration and the exchange of information between public health agencies worldwide. It enables rapid and effective coordination of efforts to prevent, control and respond to global health threats.

- **Preparing for health crises:** AI is used to simulate epidemic scenarios and assess the effectiveness of response strategies. This makes it easier to prepare for health crises and develop appropriate response plans.

With AI-based global public health surveillance, health officials can better understand global health trends, rapidly detect emerging epidemics, coordinate international public health efforts and better prepare for health crises. AI offers a unique opportunity to strengthen global public health surveillance, improve the response to global health emergencies and protect the health and well-being of populations worldwide.

Intervention and response to epidemics

Intervention and response to epidemics are essential steps in containing the spread of infectious diseases and minimising their impact on public health. The use of artificial intelligence (AI) in epidemic intervention and response offers many advantages, including early detection, efficient resource management, strategic planning and rapid coordination of public health efforts. Here's how AI is playing a key role in epidemic response and intervention:

- **Early detection of epidemics:** By analysing epidemiological data in real time, AI enables early detection of emerging epidemics. Machine learning algorithms can identify abnormal trends and unusual patterns in the data, alerting health authorities to the possibility of an epidemic in progress.

- **Resource management:** AI can help optimise resource management during an epidemic. It can predict the number of future cases, the need for hospital beds, medicines, personal protective equipment, etc., enabling health authorities to plan and distribute resources more effectively.

- **Identifying epidemic outbreaks:** AI uses geospatial analysis to identify geographical areas where epidemic outbreaks are forming. This enables public health interventions to be targeted at these high-risk areas.

- **Contact tracking:** AI can be used to track contacts of confirmed cases of an infectious disease, facilitating the rapid detection of new cases and the implementation of targeted quarantine measures.

- **Modelling the spread of the epidemic:** AI can model the spread of the epidemic using current and past epidemiological data. This enables predictions to be made about how the epidemic might develop over the coming days and weeks, helping health officials to make informed decisions.

- **Informed decision-making:** AI provides factual information and in-depth analyses to help decision-makers make informed decisions about the public health measures to be implemented to control the epidemic.

- **Communication and awareness:** AI can be used to disseminate up-to-date information on the epidemic, prevention measures and available resources. This helps to raise public awareness and encourage cooperation in the fight against the epidemic.

- **Monitoring the response:** AI makes it possible to monitor the effectiveness of public health measures implemented and provide real-time feedback to health managers, enabling response strategies to be adjusted quickly if necessary.

By combining AI with the expertise of healthcare professionals, interventions and responses to epidemics can be faster, more accurate and better adapted to the health challenges facing populations. AI offers valuable support in managing health crises and helps save lives by enabling a more effective and coordinated response to epidemics. However, it is important to note that AI is a complementary tool and does not replace human expertise in the decision-making and implementation of public health interventions.

Challenges of AI-based epidemiological surveillance

Epidemiological surveillance based on artificial intelligence (AI) offers many advantages, but it also faces significant challenges. Here are some of the main challenges of AI-based epidemiological surveillance:

- **Data quality :** Data quality is essential for effective epidemiological surveillance. AI depends on accurate, complete and reliable data to produce relevant analyses and predictions. However, epidemiological data can sometimes be incomplete, biased or erroneous, which can affect the reliability of AI results.

- **Protection of privacy:** AI-based epidemiological surveillance often involves the collection and analysis of large quantities of personal health data. It is essential to guarantee the protection of individual privacy while allowing the data to be used for public health purposes.

- **Model complexity:** AI models used for epidemiological surveillance can be complex and require specialist expertise to develop and interpret. The complexity of the models can make them difficult to use for healthcare professionals and decision-makers who are unfamiliar with AI.

- **Lack of data:** In some regions of the world, particularly in developing countries, there may be a lack of epidemiological data available to feed into AI models. This may limit the effectiveness of AI-based epidemiological surveillance in these regions.

- **Interpretability of results:** AI models, such as deep neural networks, can be difficult to interpret. It is often difficult to understand exactly how the AI has made a decision or produced a result, which can be a barrier to the acceptance and use of AI in epidemiological surveillance.

- **Financial and technological resources:** Implementing AI-based epidemiological surveillance may require significant financial and technological resources. Not all regions of the world have the necessary resources to fully adopt and deploy these technologies.
- **Integration with existing healthcare systems:** Integrating AI into existing healthcare systems can be a challenge, particularly in healthcare facilities that are not yet ready to fully embrace these new technologies.

- **Rapid response to epidemics:** While AI can help detect emerging epidemics, it is essential to be able to act quickly and effectively to control the spread of disease. AI must be used in conjunction with effective coordination of health systems and health authorities to ensure a rapid response.

Despite these challenges, the integration of AI into epidemiological surveillance offers enormous potential for improving early detection of epidemics, resource management and strategic planning. By overcoming these challenges, AI can become a valuable tool in the fight against infectious diseases and contribute to improving public health on a global scale. However, it is important to continue to evaluate and continuously improve AI-based approaches to ensure their effectiveness and usefulness in public health practice.

Preparing for future pandemics

Preparing for future pandemics is a major priority for public health officials and decision-makers around the world. Artificial intelligence (AI) plays a key role in this preparedness by enhancing capabilities for early detection, rapid response and effective resource management. Here's how AI can help prepare for future pandemics:

- **Advanced epidemiological surveillance:** AI enables advanced epidemiological surveillance by analysing epidemiological data from multiple sources in real time. By quickly identifying early warning signals, AI can help detect and predict emerging epidemics before they get out of control.

- **Predictive modelling:** AI can model the potential spread of a pandemic using historical and real-time epidemiological data. This enables decision-makers to better understand potential spread patterns and anticipate resource and response needs.

- **Scenario simulation:** AI can be used to simulate outbreak scenarios to better understand how a pandemic might evolve and what public health measures would be most effective in dealing with it. This helps develop well-informed response plans and predict the consequences of different actions.

- **Vaccine and treatment development:** AI can speed up the process of discovering and developing new vaccines and treatments by rapidly analysing large amounts of scientific data and identifying potential drug targets.

- **Monitoring international travel:** AI can monitor international travel and air travel to detect potential risks of rapid disease spread between countries. This helps to put in place border control measures to limit the spread of the pandemic.

- **Communication and awareness:** AI can be used to rapidly disseminate up-to-date information on the pandemic, prevention measures and available resources. This helps to raise public awareness and promote responsible behaviour.

- **Coordination of international efforts:** AI facilitates the international coordination of public health efforts by enabling the rapid exchange of information and data between countries. This enables a more coordinated and effective response to pandemics that cross borders.

- **Training and preparation of healthcare professionals:** AI can be used to develop online training programmes and simulations to prepare healthcare professionals to deal with a pandemic. This helps to reinforce the skills and knowledge needed to meet the challenges of a pandemic.

By preparing healthcare systems using AI and developing anticipatory response strategies, we can be better prepared to deal with future pandemics. AI offers a unique opportunity to improve pandemic preparedness, early detection and management, helping to protect public health and save lives in future health crises. However, continued investment in public health AI research and development is essential to maximise its benefits in preparing for future pandemics.

Future prospects : The evolution of epidemiological surveillance thanks to AI

The future prospects for the development of epidemiological surveillance using artificial intelligence (AI) are very promising. AI will continue to play a crucial role in the preparation, early detection, rapid response and management of future pandemics, as well as in the overall improvement of public health. Here are some key areas where AI could bring significant improvements in epidemiological surveillance:

- **Improved predictive models:** AI models used to predict the spread of epidemics will become increasingly sophisticated, taking into account more variables and risk factors. The integration of data from multiple sources, such as environmental data, social networks, wearable health sensors, etc., will enable more accurate, real-time predictions.

- **Use of unstructured data:** AI will make it possible to make better use of unstructured data, such as medical texts, images and videos, to enrich epidemiological surveillance. For example, the analysis of radiological images could help to rapidly identify specific characteristics of infectious diseases.

- **Real-time surveillance:** AI will facilitate the implementation of real-time surveillance systems, where epidemiological data is continuously collected and analysed, enabling even faster detection of emerging epidemics and a more rapid response.

- **Conversational AI and chatbots:** Conversational AI, such as chatbots, could be used to provide personalised information and advice to individuals about preventive measures, symptoms to look out for, screening centres, etc. This would help raise public awareness and answer questions quickly. This would help to raise public awareness and answer questions quickly.

- **Improved data integration:** AI will facilitate the integration of data from different healthcare systems and heterogeneous sources. This will enable a more global analysis of epidemics, identifying epidemiological trends that cross geographical and institutional boundaries.

- **Use of reinforcement learning:** Reinforcement learning could be applied to optimise public health interventions by testing different strategies and continually adjusting actions according to the results obtained.

- **Precision medicine:** AI will enable a more personalised approach to health, where individuals can benefit from health recommendations based on their genetic characteristics, medical history and lifestyle, which could help to prevent and manage disease more effectively.

- **Collective intelligence:** AI can also facilitate collaboration between public health experts around the world, enabling the rapid sharing of data, models and intervention strategies to tackle global epidemics.

However, to fully realise these future prospects, challenges must be overcome, such as data confidentiality and security, interpretability of models, acceptance by healthcare professionals and the general public, and equitable access to AI technologies worldwide. By investing in research, training and infrastructure, we can make AI a powerful tool for improving epidemiological surveillance and strengthening our ability to meet future public health challenges.

Algorithms to save lives: How AI is revolutionising medical emergencies

Introduction to medical emergencies and AI

The introduction of artificial intelligence (AI) in the field of medical emergencies promises to revolutionise the way patients are cared for in critical situations. Medical emergencies are situations where rapid and accurate medical intervention is essential to preserve the life and health of patients. AI can play a key role in improving the management of medical emergencies, providing fast and accurate assistance to healthcare professionals and improving patient outcomes. Here are some key aspects of introducing AI into medical emergencies:

- **Early detection of emergencies:** AI can be used to analyse patients' vital signs in real time, such as heart rate, blood pressure, temperature, etc., to detect early warning signs of medical distress. This enables early intervention and could help prevent serious complications.

- **Outcome prediction:** AI can be used to predict patient outcomes in emergency situations, using predictive models based on previous medical data. This can help healthcare professionals make informed decisions about treatments and interventions.
- **Diagnostic support:** AI can be used as a diagnostic support tool in medical emergencies by analysing patient data and providing suggestions on the possible causes of presenting symptoms. This can help doctors make a diagnosis more quickly and accurately.

126

- **Optimising triage:** AI can be used to optimise patient triage in emergency departments, identifying the most critical patients who require immediate attention and helping to allocate resources according to severity.

- **Assistance with medical procedures:** AI can be used to help doctors with complex medical procedures, such as intubation or catheter placement, by providing real-time information on the position and orientation of medical instruments.

- **Decision support:** AI can be used to provide recommendations to doctors based on specific patient data and best medical practice. This can help doctors make quick and informed decisions during emergencies.

- **Training and simulation:** AI can be used to develop simulations of medical emergencies, enabling healthcare professionals to practise managing critical situations in a safe, controlled environment.

- **Communication and coordination:** AI can facilitate communication and coordination between the various members of the medical team during emergencies, by providing real-time information on the patient's condition and the actions being taken.

The introduction of AI into medical emergencies has the potential to transform the way we manage emergency situations and improve patient care when they need it most. However, it is important to note that AI does not replace healthcare professionals, but assists and supports them in their decision-making and emergency management. AI is a powerful tool that, used responsibly, can significantly improve the quality of emergency care and save lives.

Early detection of medical emergencies

Early detection of medical emergencies is a crucial aspect of healthcare, enabling rapid and appropriate intervention to preserve the life and health of patients. The introduction of artificial intelligence (AI) in this area has the potential to significantly improve the early detection of medical emergencies by analysing patient data in real time and identifying early warning signals. Here are some of the ways AI can contribute to the early detection of medical emergencies:

- **Analysis of vital signs:** AI can analyse patients' vital signs, such as heart rate, blood pressure, temperature and oxygen saturation, in real time. It can detect abnormal variations in vital signs that could indicate a critical condition, enabling rapid intervention.

- **Continuous data processing:** AI is capable of continuously processing large quantities of data from medical monitors, wearable sensors and other sources. This enables continuous monitoring of patients, which is essential for rapidly detecting changes in their state of health.

- **Predictive modelling:** AI can use predictive models based on previous medical data to anticipate the risk of complications or deterioration in a given patient. This helps healthcare professionals to take preventive measures to avoid emergencies.

- **Trend detection:** AI can detect long-term trends in patient data, such as a gradual deterioration in their state of health. This early detection of gradual changes can be crucial in preventing medical emergencies.

- **Complex pattern identification:** AI can identify complex and subtle patterns in patient data that could indicate an impending emergency. These patterns can be difficult for humans to detect, but AI can identify them quickly.

- **Integration of heterogeneous data:** AI can integrate heterogeneous data from different sources, including electronic medical records, medical images and genetic information. This holistic approach helps to better understand a patient's state of health and anticipate potential risks.
- **Preventive alerts:** AI can generate preventive alerts for healthcare professionals when a patient's data indicates imminent deterioration. This enables doctors and nurses to intervene quickly and provide emergency care before the situation worsens.

- **Using real-time data:** AI can use real-time data to detect medical emergencies as soon as they occur. This is particularly important in emergency situations where every minute counts.

By integrating AI into the early detection of medical emergencies, healthcare professionals can benefit from valuable assistance in making rapid and informed decisions. This can save lives and improve patient outcomes in critical situations. However, it is important to note that AI must be used responsibly and in conjunction with human medical expertise, as it cannot replace the clinical judgement of healthcare professionals.

Sorting and allocating resources

Triage and resource allocation are essential elements in the management of medical emergencies, particularly in crisis situations where resources may be limited. The introduction of artificial intelligence (AI) in this area offers opportunities to improve the efficiency and accuracy of triage, as well as to optimise resource allocation to meet patient needs more effectively. Here's how AI can contribute to triage and resource allocation:

- **Early and accurate triage:** AI can help to quickly and accurately assess the severity of patients as soon as they arrive at A&E. By analysing patients' vital signs, symptoms and medical history, AI can classify patients according to their level of urgency and priority for treatment.

- **Personalised triage algorithms:** AI can use personalised triage algorithms that take into account the individual characteristics of each patient to assess the severity of their condition. This allows triage to be tailored to each patient's specific needs.

- **Severity prediction:** AI can predict the likely severity of a patient's condition based on previous medical data and predictive models. This enables healthcare professionals to make informed decisions about resource allocation by anticipating future needs.

- **Optimising resources:** AI can help to optimise the allocation of resources according to the severity of cases. For example, it can help determine which patients require immediate hospitalisation, which patients can be treated on an outpatient basis and which patients can be cared for at home.

- **Fairness in resource allocation:** AI can be used to ensure that resources are allocated fairly, taking into account the needs of all patients, regardless of their social origin, race or economic status.

- **Bed availability management:** AI can help manage the availability of hospital beds in real time, forecasting future needs and optimising patient flows to avoid bottlenecks.

- **Predicting the resources needed:** AI can predict the medical resources needed based on the severity of cases and epidemiological trends. This enables proactive planning and efficient use of resources.

- **Dynamic reallocation of resources:** AI can help with the dynamic reallocation of resources according to the changing needs of patients. For example, it can help reallocate medical staff or equipment in real time to respond to critical emergencies.

By using AI for triage and resource allocation, healthcare institutions can improve patient management in emergency situations, optimise the use of limited resources and improve clinical outcomes. However, it is important to note that AI must be used responsibly and ethically, bearing in mind that the final decision must always be made by healthcare professionals taking into account the specific context and condition of the patient. AI is a powerful tool that, when used wisely, can help improve healthcare in emergency situations.

Improving the effectiveness of emergency protocols

The introduction of artificial intelligence (AI) into medical emergency protocols promises to significantly improve their efficiency, which can translate into better clinical outcomes for patients and better use of medical resources. Here's how AI can help improve the efficiency of emergency protocols:

- **Rapid data analysis:** AI can rapidly analyse large amounts of data from multiple sources, including patient vital signs, laboratory test results, medical images and electronic medical records. Using sophisticated algorithms, AI can extract relevant information in real time, enabling a rapid assessment of a patient's condition.

- **Diagnostic assistance:** AI can provide valuable assistance to doctors by suggesting possible diagnoses based on patient data and the symptoms presented. This saves doctors time in making a diagnosis and enables them to start appropriate treatment quickly.

- **Informed decision-making:** Using predictive models based on past medical data, AI can help doctors make informed decisions about treatments and interventions. This optimises patient care.

- **Optimised triage:** AI can help to optimise the triage of patients as soon as they arrive at A&E by quickly assessing the seriousness of their condition. This allows resources to be allocated according to the urgency of each case, improving the overall efficiency of patient care.

- **Assistance during medical procedures:** AI can be used as an aid during complex medical procedures, such as intubation or surgery, by providing real-time information on the position and orientation of medical instruments.

- **Bed availability management:** AI can predict future hospital bed requirements based on epidemiological trends and patient data. This enables better management of bed availability and optimisation of patient flows.

- **Early detection of complications:** AI can detect early warning signs of complications in patients, enabling rapid intervention to prevent more serious health problems.

- **Simulation and training:** AI can be used to develop simulations of medical emergencies, enabling healthcare professionals to train in the management of critical situations in a safe, controlled environment. This improves their responsiveness and preparedness in real emergency situations.

By improving the efficiency of emergency protocols, AI can help save lives and improve patient outcomes in critical situations. However, it is important to note that AI does not replace healthcare professionals, but assists and supports them in their decision-making and emergency management. AI is a powerful tool that, when used responsibly and in conjunction with human medical expertise, can significantly improve the quality of emergency care.

Integration of AI technologies in ambulances

Integrating artificial intelligence (AI) technologies into ambulances can transform the delivery of emergency care by improving early detection of medical emergencies, providing assistance to healthcare professionals and optimising the use of medical resources. Here's how AI can be integrated into ambulances to improve emergency care:

- **Real-time monitoring:** Ambulances equipped with real-time medical monitoring devices can collect patients' vital signs and transmit this data to an AI system. The AI can analyse this data in real time to detect early signs of medical distress and alert the medical team in an emergency.

- **Diagnostic support:** AI can be used as a diagnostic support tool in ambulances. By analysing patient data, AI can provide suggestions for possible diagnoses and treatment recommendations, helping healthcare professionals to make informed decisions during patient transport.

- **Optimised triage:** AI can help to optimise patient triage as soon as they are picked up in the ambulance. By quickly assessing the seriousness of patients, AI can help the medical team to allocate resources appropriately, prioritising the most critical patients for transport to the right healthcare facilities.

- **Real-time information transfer:** AI can facilitate the transmission of important information between the ambulance and the destination healthcare facility. For example, AI can inform the hospital's medical team of the patient's condition and the interventions already carried out in the ambulance, enabling smoother care on arrival at the hospital.

- **Guidance during medical procedures:** AI can be used to provide real-time information to healthcare professionals during emergency medical procedures, such as intubation or drug administration. This can help improve the accuracy and safety of these critical procedures.

- **Predicting resource requirements:** AI can predict the medical resources needed for each emergency, enabling better planning of patient transport and reception in healthcare establishments.

- **Training and simulation:** AI can be used to develop simulations of medical emergencies in ambulances, enabling healthcare professionals to practise managing critical situations in a safe, controlled environment.

Integrating AI technologies into ambulances can help improve emergency care by enabling faster detection of medical emergencies, providing assistance to healthcare professionals during interventions and optimising the use of medical resources. However, it is essential to ensure that these technologies are used responsibly and ethically, bearing in mind that AI must always be complementary to the expertise and clinical judgement of healthcare professionals. AI offers considerable potential to improve emergency care and save lives, but it must be used with caution and with respect for ethical principles and patient safety.

Challenges and limits of using AI in medical emergencies

The use of artificial intelligence (AI) in medical emergencies offers many benefits, but it also faces a number of challenges and limitations that need to be considered for safe and effective implementation. Some of the key challenges and limitations include:

- **Data reliability:** AI relies on accurate and reliable data to make informed decisions. If incoming data is incomplete, erroneous or biased, this can lead to errors in AI predictions and recommendations, which can have serious consequences in emergency situations.

- **Complexity of emergency situations:** Medical emergencies can be complex and varied, and each patient is unique. AI can sometimes struggle to manage the diversity of cases and provide appropriate recommendations in unusual or unexpected situations.

- **Accountability and decision-making:** Although AI can provide suggestions and predictions based on past data, the ultimate responsibility for decision-making still lies with healthcare professionals. Doctors must therefore be able to understand the reasons behind AI recommendations and make informed decisions taking into account the specific clinical context.

- **Integration into clinical workflows:** Integrating AI into medical emergencies can require significant changes to existing clinical workflows. It can be challenging to adopt new technologies and ensure they work seamlessly with existing healthcare systems.

- **Data security:** The use of AI in medical emergencies involves the collection, storage and processing of large amounts of sensitive patient data. It is essential to ensure that this data is secure and protected against privacy breaches and cyber attacks.

- **Training and skills:** Healthcare professionals must be properly trained in the use of AI and the interpretation of results. Adequate training is essential to ensure the appropriate use of AI in medical emergencies.

- **Ethics and responsibility:** AI raises ethical issues, particularly with regard to autonomous decision-making and responsibility in the event of errors. It is essential to ensure that the decisions taken by AI are transparent, understandable and fair.

- **Cost and accessibility:** Integrating AI into medical emergencies can represent a significant financial investment. It is important to ensure that these technologies are affordable and accessible to all healthcare establishments, including those with limited resources.

In conclusion, the use of AI in medical emergencies offers many opportunities to improve patient care and optimise the use of medical resources. However, it is essential to address the challenges and consider the limitations of this technology to ensure responsible and safe implementation. AI should be used as a complementary tool to support healthcare professionals and improve clinical decisions, but it should never replace clinical judgement and human medical expertise.

Outlook for the future :
The evolution of medical emergencies thanks to AI

The prospects for the future use of artificial intelligence (AI) in medical emergencies are very promising. AI continues to advance rapidly, and its integration into emergency care is set to radically transform the way we manage and respond to medical emergencies. Here are some of the key prospects for the future of AI in medical emergencies:

- **Improved early detection:** AI will continue to play a key role in the early detection of medical emergencies by analysing patient data in real time, identifying early warning signals and quickly alerting healthcare professionals. This will enable faster and more effective intervention to save lives.

- **Personalised care:** AI will evolve to provide personalised recommendations and treatments based on the individual characteristics of each patient. Through the use of machine learning and genetic data, AI will be able to predict patient response to certain treatments and adapt protocols accordingly.

- **Full integration of medical data:** AI will facilitate the full integration of medical data from a variety of sources, including electronic medical records, medical devices, wearable sensors and genomic data. This will enable a more holistic view of patient health and better clinical decision-making.

- **Strengthening medical training:** AI will continue to be used for medical simulation and training, enabling healthcare professionals to train in realistic, risk-free emergency scenarios. This will improve their responsiveness and preparedness when faced with real-life emergencies.

- **Telemedicine and remote assistance:** AI will enable an expansion of telemedicine in emergency situations, providing assistance to healthcare professionals in remote or underserved areas. AI systems will be able to help diagnose and manage medical emergencies remotely.

- **Preventing emergencies:** By analysing health data in real time, AI will be able to help prevent medical emergencies by identifying risk factors in patients and taking appropriate preventive measures.

- **Integration of robots in emergency departments:** Intelligent nursing robots and autonomous devices can be integrated into medical emergency departments to provide additional assistance to medical teams and help manage patients.

- **Evolution of emergency protocols:** AI will continue to evolve to improve the efficiency of emergency protocols, optimising triage, resource management and clinical decisions.

However, it is important to note that the introduction of AI into medical emergencies must be accompanied by ethical considerations, appropriate regulations and patient safety guarantees. Responsible and ethical use of AI is essential to maximise its benefits and minimise potential risks.

In conclusion, AI offers enormous potential to improve medical emergencies, enabling early detection, informed decision-making and effective resource management. Its progressive integration into emergency care promises to improve clinical outcomes, save lives and transform the way we respond to medical emergencies.

AI in medical research: revolutionary discoveries and new horizons

Introduction to AI in medical research

The introduction of artificial intelligence (AI) into medical research has opened up new perspectives and significantly transformed the way scientists approach the discovery of new knowledge in medicine. AI offers powerful tools for analysing, interpreting and drawing conclusions from large medical datasets, speeding up the research process and paving the way for new medical breakthroughs. Here is an introduction to the main aspects of AI in medical research:

- **Machine learning and data analysis:** Machine learning is a branch of AI that allows computers to learn from data without being explicitly programmed. In medical research, machine learning can be used to analyse large amounts of medical data, such as medical images, genomic sequences or electronic medical records, to identify hidden patterns and relationships. This speeds up data analysis and identifies new associations between biological factors and diseases.

- **Biomarker discovery:** AI enables researchers to discover new biomarkers, i.e. specific biological indicators that can be used to diagnose, predict or monitor the course of a disease. By analysing large patient datasets, AI can identify relevant biomarkers that can improve the accuracy of diagnosis and prognosis.

- **Disease diagnosis and prediction:** AI can be used to develop predictive models capable of diagnosing and predicting diseases. Using machine learning algorithms, AI can analyse patients' symptoms, medical history and risk factors to provide faster and more accurate diagnoses.

- **Drug development:** AI can accelerate the drug development process by identifying potential therapeutic targets and predicting drug efficacy based on genomic and pharmacological data. This optimises drug design and reduces research costs.

- **Precision medicine:** AI plays a key role in precision medicine by enabling treatments to be tailored to individual patient characteristics. By analysing genetic profiles, medical data and responses to treatment, AI can recommend more targeted and effective therapies.

- **Medical imaging research:** AI is widely used in the analysis of medical images, such as X-rays, MRIs and scans. Machine learning algorithms can help to automatically detect and identify anomalies, enabling radiologists and doctors to make faster and more accurate decisions.

- **Clinical trial management:** AI can be used to optimise the design and management of clinical trials, by identifying appropriate patient populations for trials, monitoring drug safety and analysing trial results.

In short, AI offers vast possibilities in the field of medical research by speeding up the processes of analysis, discovery and decision-making. It is helping to advance medicine by paving the way for new discoveries, more accurate diagnoses and more effective treatments. However, it is important to stress that AI must be used responsibly and ethically, always bearing in mind that medical research must be guided by ethical values and patient safety principles.

Analysis of massive data in medical research

The analysis of massive data, also known as 'Big Data', is playing a key role in medical research thanks to the integration of artificial intelligence (AI) and machine learning. Advances in technology and access to vast medical datasets have opened up new vistas for medical research, enabling scientists to better understand diseases, discover new treatments and personalise healthcare. Here's how massive data analysis is being used in medical research:

- **Discovering patterns and correlations:** Massive data analytics can identify hidden patterns and correlations in vast medical datasets. Researchers can analyse multiple variables, such as symptoms, risk factors, test results, medical history and genetic data, to find significant relationships between different factors and diseases.

- **Disease prediction and prevention:** By analysing massive amounts of data, researchers can develop predictive models that make it possible to anticipate the risk of developing certain diseases in individuals. This enables a preventive approach to health by identifying people at high risk and offering them targeted interventions to prevent the development of disease.

- **Precision medicine:** Massive data analysis makes it possible to tailor treatments to individual patient characteristics. By analysing patients' genetic data and medical profiles, researchers can identify the most appropriate treatments for each individual, thereby improving the effectiveness of therapies.

- **Identification of biomarkers:** Massive data analysis can help to identify new biomarkers, i.e. specific biological indicators associated with certain diseases. These biomarkers can be used to diagnose diseases earlier, monitor disease progression and assess the effectiveness of treatments.

- **Medical imaging research:** Medical images, such as scans, MRIs and X-rays, generate vast quantities of data. Analysing these large-scale images using AI can automatically identify anomalies, facilitate diagnosis and improve patient care.

- **Optimising clinical trials:** Massive data analysis can be used to optimise the design and management of clinical trials. Researchers can rapidly identify appropriate patient populations for trials, improve participant selection and analyse results more efficiently.

- **Public health and epidemiology:** Massive data analysis is essential for epidemiological surveillance, enabling the early detection of epidemics, predictive modelling of infectious diseases and the implementation of effective public health measures.

In conclusion, massive data analysis is an essential component of modern medical research, allowing researchers to leverage AI and machine learning to extract valuable information from vast medical datasets. This revolutionary approach is helping to advance medicine by enabling a deeper understanding of disease, personalised care and improved overall patient outcomes. However, it is important to ensure that this analysis is carried out responsibly, ethically and in compliance with medical data confidentiality standards.

Discovering personalised medicines and therapies

Artificial intelligence (AI) is playing an increasingly important role in drug discovery and the development of personalised therapies. Thanks to its ability to analyse data rapidly and in depth, AI is speeding up the research process and enabling a more targeted approach to the development of treatments. Here's how AI is being used in drug discovery and personalised therapies:

- **Virtual drug screening:** One of the most promising uses of AI in drug discovery is virtual screening. AI can analyse vast databases of chemical compounds to identify those most likely to bind to a specific target, such as a protein involved in a disease. This approach enables the rapid identification of potential candidates for new drugs, considerably reducing the time and costs associated with the search for new molecules.

- **Searching for therapeutic targets:** AI can be used to analyse complex datasets, such as genomic or proteomic data, to identify new therapeutic targets. This provides a better understanding of the underlying mechanisms of disease and identifies potential biological pathways for the development of treatments.

- **Personalised treatments:** AI makes it possible to develop personalised therapies by analysing patients' individual characteristics, such as their genetic profile, medical history and response to certain treatments. Using this information, AI can recommend treatments tailored to each patient, improving the effectiveness of therapies and reducing undesirable side effects.

- **Optimising clinical trials:** AI can be used to optimise the design and management of clinical trials for new drugs. By analysing clinical trial data, AI can identify patient populations most likely to benefit from treatment and improve participant selection, speeding up the drug development process.

- **Detecting new uses for existing drugs:** AI can help identify new uses for existing drugs by analysing large clinical datasets. For example, some drugs may have unexpected benefits in treating diseases other than those for which they were originally developed.

- **Optimising drug formulations:** AI can also be used to optimise drug formulations, finding the most effective dosages and appropriate routes of administration for each patient.

In conclusion, artificial intelligence offers exciting opportunities in drug discovery and the development of personalised therapies. Through the rapid and in-depth analysis of data, AI is enabling a more targeted and effective approach to the development of treatments for diseases. However, it is important to stress that AI does not replace the role of scientists and researchers, but rather acts as a powerful tool to accelerate the research process and open up new perspectives in the fight against disease. Responsible use of AI, in line with ethical standards and regulations, is essential to ensure that its benefits are fully exploited in the field of medicine.

Human-machine collaboration in medical research

Human-machine collaboration in medical research, also known as 'augmented intelligence', is an approach in which artificial intelligence (AI) and humans work together to solve complex problems in medicine. This approach capitalises on the distinct advantages of both parties, making it possible to significantly improve the efficiency and accuracy of medical research processes. Here's how this collaboration works and its benefits:

- **Massive data processing:** AI excels at processing large amounts of medical data, but humans are essential for interpreting the results and making informed decisions. By collaborating with AI, researchers can exploit its ability to rapidly analyse large datasets and detect complex patterns, while they can bring their expertise to interpret the results and put them into a medical context.

- **Identifying new avenues of research:** AI can be used to identify new therapeutic targets, relevant biomarkers and complex relationships between genetic and environmental factors and disease. This information can then be used by human researchers to design targeted studies and further research in these promising areas.

- **Optimising clinical trials:** AI can help optimise clinical trials by identifying the most appropriate patient populations for trials, designing effective protocols and monitoring results. Human researchers can then supervise the trials, make ethical decisions and interpret the final results.

- **Drug and therapy development:** AI can speed up the process of drug screening and therapy discovery by analysing vast databases of chemical compounds and medical data. Human researchers play an essential role in the design and validation of these treatments, guaranteeing their safety and efficacy.

- **Precision medicine:** AI makes it possible to tailor treatments to individual patient characteristics. AI predictive models can help identify the most appropriate treatments for each patient based on their genetic profile, medical history and response to certain treatments. Healthcare professionals can then refine these recommendations based on their clinical experience and judgement.

- **Early detection of disease:** AI can help detect early signals of certain diseases, enabling faster diagnosis and early intervention. Human researchers can use this information to develop targeted screening programmes and devise appropriate treatment plans.

In short, human-machine collaboration in medical research is a win-win approach that capitalises on the strengths of each party to tackle the complex challenges of medicine. AI provides powerful tools for analysing massive data, discovering new knowledge and optimising processes, while human researchers contribute their clinical expertise, ethical judgement and intuition to transform these results into concrete medical advances. By working hand in hand, AI and humans are opening up new perspectives in medical research and the medicine of tomorrow. However, it is crucial to ensure the responsible use of AI by guaranteeing the confidentiality of medical data, complying with ethical standards and taking into account the limits of AI to ensure the safety and well-being of patients.

Forging an integrated future of AI and humanity in healthcare

Forging an integrated future of artificial intelligence (AI) and humanity in healthcare is essential to maximise the benefits of technology while preserving the essence of human-centred medicine. This intelligent integration is based on the idea that AI should not replace humans, but rather act as a powerful and complementary partner in the delivery of healthcare. Here are some key points to forge this integrated future:

- **Humanity at the heart of care:** Despite technological advances, compassion, empathy and human communication remain essential elements of the carer-patient relationship. AI can relieve administrative and repetitive tasks, allowing carers to devote more time to listening to patients, building relationships and providing compassionate care.

- **Training and education:** It is essential to integrate AI into the training programmes of healthcare professionals. Future carers need to be trained to work fluidly with AI systems, interpret results, make informed decisions and maintain a strong sense of ethics in using the technology.

- **Collaboration between AI and carers:** Carers need to be involved in the development and implementation of healthcare AI solutions. Their knowledge and perspectives are essential to ensure that the technology meets the real needs of patients and medical staff.

- **Ethics and data privacy:** A strong ethical framework is essential to guide the use of AI in healthcare. Protecting patient privacy and ensuring the security of medical data is paramount, while ensuring that AI-based decisions are transparent, explainable and fair.

- **Personalised care:** AI can enable a more personalised approach to care by analysing individual patient data. However, it is essential that this personalisation is guided by patients' wishes and preferences, respecting their autonomy and right to make informed decisions.

- **Equitable access to care:** AI can help to improve access to healthcare by eliminating certain geographical barriers and optimising the management of resources. However, it is important to ensure that these technologies benefit everyone, including disadvantaged and under-represented populations.

- **Validation and regulation:** Any AI technology used in medicine must be rigorously validated and regulated to ensure its effectiveness and safety. Regulatory bodies play a crucial role in setting high quality standards for the use of AI in healthcare.

By combining human expertise with the power of AI, it is possible to create a more efficient, accurate and patient-centred healthcare system. Carers can use AI to underpin their clinical skills, speed up diagnosis and treatment, and deliver more personalised and informed care. AI can also enable better resource management and more efficient use of medical data, paving the way for more predictive and preventative medicine.

However, it is important to recognise that AI is not a miracle solution and must be used with care. Mistakes can happen, and humans must always play a supervisory and validating role. The future of AI-enabled healthcare lies in the responsible, ethical and thoughtful use of technology, always bearing in mind that the ultimate goal is to improve the health and well-being of patients while preserving the essence of the carer-patient relationship.

From analysing symptoms to prescribing: How AI is reinventing the front line of care

The evolution of the front line of healthcare

The evolution of primary care is closely linked to advances in technology, medical innovation and the changing needs of patients. The front line of healthcare is the point of entry into the healthcare system for patients, where they usually meet healthcare professionals such as GPs, nurses, pharmacists and other front-line healthcare professionals. Here are some key aspects of the evolution of primary care:

- **Technology and telemedicine:** Technological advances, including artificial intelligence and mobile health applications, have made it possible to provide more effective and accessible healthcare. Telemedicine allows patients to consult their healthcare professionals remotely, which is particularly beneficial for people living in remote areas or with mobility difficulties.

- **Rapid and accurate   diagnoses:** Advances in diagnostic technologies have made it possible to speed up and improve the diagnostic process. New screening tools, biomarkers and medical imaging allow health problems to be identified earlier, leading to more effective treatments and improved outcomes.
- **Personalised care:** The evolution of the front line of healthcare includes a more personalised approach to care, taking into account the unique characteristics of each patient. Advances in genomics and precision

medicine are enabling healthcare professionals to offer treatments tailored to patients' genetic characteristics and individual preferences.

- **Prevention and health promotion:** The front line of healthcare is increasingly focused on disease prevention and health promotion. Health professionals work with patients to adopt a healthy lifestyle, detect risk factors and prevent illness before it becomes serious.

- **Integration of care:** The evolution of the front line of healthcare promotes an integrated and coordinated approach to care. Healthcare professionals work together and with other specialists to provide comprehensive and holistic care to patients.

- **Patient empowerment:** Patients are increasingly involved in their medical care. Healthcare professionals encourage patients to participate actively in decision-making about their health and to play an active role in managing their condition.

- **Collaborating with new technologies:** Frontline healthcare professionals are increasingly being trained to use new technologies, including AI systems and digital tools, to improve their practice and deliver more effective care.

- **Improved access to care:** The evolution of the front line of healthcare aims to improve access to care for all patients, with a focus on equity and universal coverage.

In short, the evolution of the front line of healthcare aims to provide more effective, personalised, preventive and accessible care for patients. Technological advances, personalised care, disease prevention and patient involvement are all factors contributing to this positive evolution. By remaining at the forefront of medical innovation and adopting a patient-centred approach, the front line of healthcare will continue to play a crucial role in improving the health of individuals and communities.

AI for symptom analysis

The use of artificial intelligence (AI) to analyse symptoms is one of the most promising advances in healthcare. AI can play a vital role in the rapid and accurate assessment of symptoms, enabling healthcare professionals to make earlier diagnoses and offer treatments tailored to patients' individual needs. Here's how AI is being used for symptom analysis:

- **Massive data analysis:** AI is capable of analysing huge amounts of medical data from a variety of sources, such as electronic health records, medical publications, clinical studies and even genomic data. This allows AI systems to identify correlations and patterns that would be difficult for humans to detect on their own.

- **Machine learning:** AI uses machine learning algorithms to learn from data and continually improve its performance. As the AI receives more data, it becomes more accurate in its analysis of symptoms and diagnoses.

- **Diagnostic prediction:** By analysing symptoms, medical history and other relevant data, AI can provide likely diagnostic assessments. This helps healthcare professionals establish treatment plans more quickly and in a more targeted way.

- **Early detection of disease:** AI can help detect subtle symptoms that could indicate a developing disease, even before obvious symptoms appear. This paves the way for earlier preventive interventions to improve health outcomes.

- **Clinical decision support:** AI can support healthcare professionals by providing additional information on symptoms and suggesting treatment options based on current best medical practice.

- **Emergency triage:** In medical emergencies, AI can help to triage patients according to the severity of their symptoms, helping to prioritise the most critical cases and reduce waiting times.

- **Chronic disease monitoring and management:** AI can continuously monitor the symptoms of patients with chronic diseases and alert healthcare professionals to significant changes, enabling proactive disease management.

- **Improved medical research:** AI can be used to analyse large-scale clinical and genomic data to identify new links between symptoms, diseases and responses to treatments. This paves the way for new medical discoveries and more personalised medicine.

It is important to note that AI for symptom analysis is designed to complement the clinical judgement of healthcare professionals, not replace it. AI systems are powerful tools, but they must be used responsibly and ethically to ensure optimal outcomes and patient safety. In combination with human expertise, AI can revolutionise the way symptoms are assessed, diagnosed and treated, leading to more effective and personalised healthcare.

AI-assisted diagnostics

Artificial Intelligence (AI)-assisted diagnosis is an approach that combines the clinical expertise of healthcare professionals with the power of AI to improve the accuracy and speed of medical diagnoses. The aim is to provide a more accurate diagnostic assessment by using machine learning algorithms to analyse medical data and propose likely diagnostic assessments.

Here's how AI-assisted diagnosis works:

- **Collecting medical data:** Healthcare professionals collect relevant medical data, such as patient symptoms, medical history, results of medical examinations, laboratory tests, medical images, etc.

- **Integration of data into the AI system:** Medical data is integrated into the AI system, which uses machine learning algorithms to analyse the information and detect patterns and correlations.

- **Analysing data and proposing diagnoses:** AI analyses data using predictive models developed from a large number of similar medical cases. On the basis of this analysis, AI proposes probable diagnostic assessments that help healthcare professionals to guide their research and investigations.

- **Shared decision-making:** Healthcare professionals use the diagnostic assessments proposed by AI as a complementary resource in their clinical decision-making process. They discuss diagnostic options with patients and make informed decisions based on the clinical expertise and information provided by AI.

- **Continuous improvement:** The AI system is continually improving as it receives more data and feedback from healthcare professionals. The more it is used, the more the AI can refine its predictive models and become more accurate in its diagnostic assessments.

AI-assisted diagnosis has a number of important advantages:
- **Improved accuracy:** AI can help detect subtle relationships between symptoms, medical history and diagnoses, improving the accuracy of diagnostic assessments.

- **Speed:** AI can analyse large quantities of data in a very short space of time, enabling faster and more effective diagnostic assessment.

- **Access to expertise:** In certain regions where access to medical specialists is limited, AI-assisted diagnosis can provide healthcare professionals with rapid access to expertise and advanced medical knowledge.

- **Personalised care:** AI can help identify unique individual characteristics in patients, enabling more personalised medical care tailored to their specific needs.

However, it is essential to note that AI-assisted diagnosis does not replace the expertise and clinical experience of healthcare professionals. Rather, it is a complementary tool designed to improve clinical decision-making and provide probable diagnostic assessments to support the work of physicians and other healthcare professionals. Responsible and ethical use of AI in diagnosis is essential to ensure high quality care and patient safety.

Predicting disease progression

Predicting the progression of disease is an area of medical research in which artificial intelligence (AI) plays a crucial role. The aim is to use sophisticated AI models to anticipate the progression of a disease in a patient, based on their individual characteristics, medical history and other relevant factors. This approach offers a number of advantages for patient management and healthcare planning.

Here's how AI predicts disease progression:

- **Data collection:** Patient medical data, such as laboratory test results, medical images, medical history and symptoms, are collected and used as input for the AI models.

- **Predictive modelling:** AI models, based on machine learning, are trained on a large set of patient data to identify patterns and risk factors associated with disease progression. The more data the model receives, the more accurate its predictions become.

- **Identification of risk factors:** AI models identify specific risk factors that are linked to faster or slower disease progression in the patient. These factors may include specific biomarkers, levels of certain biological markers, health behaviours, etc.

- **Progression predictions:** Once the AI model has been trained, it is used to make predictions about the future progression of the patient's disease. This can include estimates of symptom progression, possible complications and expected treatment efficacy.

- **Care planning:** Predictions of disease progression help healthcare professionals to proactively plan care.

They can develop personalised treatment plans based on the predictions, enabling more effective disease management.

The areas of application for disease progression prediction are varied and include chronic diseases such as diabetes, heart disease, cancer, Alzheimer's disease, multiple sclerosis, among others. Here are some important benefits of using AI to predict disease progression:

- **Early detection of complications:** Predicting disease progression means that potential complications can be detected earlier in patients, facilitating preventive intervention.

- **Personalised treatment:** Progression predictions help to tailor treatments to individual patient characteristics, which can improve treatment effectiveness.

- **Resource management:** Disease progression forecasts help to plan the use of healthcare resources more effectively, by identifying patients who may need more intensive care.

- **Better communication with patients:** Progression predictions can help healthcare professionals communicate more effectively with patients about their condition and treatment options.

- **Advances in research:** Using AI to predict the progression of diseases can also contribute to the advancement of medical research by identifying new risk factors and opening up new avenues of research.

However, it is important to note that the prediction of disease progression is still a developing field, and certain limitations must be taken into account. AI models are not infallible and can be influenced by biases in the training data. In addition, the complexity of diseases and the interconnectedness of many factors can make prediction of progression difficult. It is therefore essential to use AI responsibly and combine predictions with clinical expertise to make informed healthcare decisions.

Personalised prescription and follow-up

Personalised prescribing and monitoring using artificial intelligence (AI) represents a major advance in healthcare. This approach aims to provide medical treatments tailored to the individual characteristics of each patient, using machine learning algorithms to analyse medical data and generate tailored treatment recommendations. Here's how personalised prescribing and monitoring with the help of AI works:

- **Collection of medical data:** Healthcare professionals collect detailed medical data on patients, such as their medical history, symptoms, laboratory test results, medical images, genetic profile, lifestyle and other relevant factors.

- **Data analysis:** Patient medical data is analysed by AI models powered by machine learning algorithms. These models examine individual patient characteristics and compare them to large datasets of similar patients to detect patterns and correlations.

- **Treatment recommendations:** Based on the results of the analysis, the AI generates personalised treatment recommendations for the patient. These recommendations can include specific drug choices, dosages, treatment durations and complementary therapies tailored to the patient's unique needs.

- **Continuous monitoring:** Once treatment has been prescribed, AI can be used to continuously monitor the patient's progress. Monitoring data, such as responses to treatment, side effects, symptom changes and other information, is fed into the AI system to adjust treatment recommendations over time.

- **Reassessment and improvement:** As new data is collected and the patient's treatment progresses, the AI regularly reassesses the recommendations to ensure that they are still tailored to the patient's needs. The AI is continually improving as it receives more data and feedback.

The benefits of personalised prescribing and monitoring thanks to AI are numerous:

- **Customised treatment:** Personalised treatments respond to the specific characteristics of each patient, increasing their efficacy and safety.

- **Reducing errors:** AI can help avoid prescribing errors due to potentially dangerous drug interactions or inappropriate dosages.

- **Chronic disease management:** for patients suffering from chronic diseases, AI can continuously monitor their state of health and adjust treatments according to their progress.
- **Optimising results:** Personalised treatments aim to optimise clinical results and improve patients' quality of life.

- **Preventing recurrences:** By identifying individual risk factors, AI can help prevent recurrences of disease or complications.

However, it is important to note that personalised prescribing and monitoring with the help of AI does not replace the expertise and clinical experience of healthcare professionals. AI is designed to complement their judgement and knowledge, not replace it. Close collaboration between healthcare professionals and AI is essential to ensure high-quality care and to make informed treatment decisions. Therefore, responsible and ethical use of AI is essential to maximise its benefits in personalised prescribing and monitoring.

Telemedicine and virtual assistance

Telemedicine and virtual assistance are rapidly expanding areas of healthcare, made possible by advances in artificial intelligence (AI) and communications technology. These revolutionary approaches enable healthcare professionals to provide care and medical advice remotely, using virtual platforms and sophisticated AI systems. Here's how telemedicine and virtual assistance work:

1. Telemedicine :
Telemedicine is the provision of healthcare services at a distance using communication technologies such as video calls, secure messaging or mobile applications. AI plays a key role in telemedicine by improving communication between healthcare professionals and patients, facilitating the sharing of medical data and providing real-time analysis.

- **Virtual consultations:** Patients can consult doctors or specialists remotely through virtual consultations using secure videoconferencing platforms. AI can help match the patient with the appropriate healthcare professional based on the patient's symptoms and medical history.

- **Remote medical monitoring:** Patients suffering from chronic illnesses can benefit from regular medical monitoring without having to travel frequently. AI can help to continuously monitor patients' health data and alert healthcare professionals to any significant changes.

- **Remote diagnosis:** In some remote or underserved areas, telemedicine can enable patients to access specialist diagnostic services without leaving their geographical area. AI can support remote diagnosis by analysing medical images or providing likely diagnostic assessments.

2. Virtual assistance :

AI-powered virtual assistants are also playing an important role in healthcare by providing automated and personalised assistance to patients and healthcare professionals.

- **Answers to patients' questions:** Virtual assistants can provide answers to patients' common questions about symptoms, medicines, medical procedures, etc. This enables patients to obtain information quickly and in a personalised way.

- **Appointment management:** Virtual assistants can manage medical appointments, send reminders to patients and make it easier to schedule medical visits.

- **Patient education:** Virtual assistants can provide educational information on diseases, treatments, lifestyle changes and other health-related aspects.

This helps to empower patients and improve their understanding of their own health.

- **Medical data analysis:** virtual assistants can analyse patients' medical data and provide healthcare professionals with recommendations for personalised treatment plans.

Telemedicine and virtual assistance offer many advantages:
- **Accessibility:** Telemedicine increases access to healthcare, particularly in remote or underserved areas, and for patients with reduced mobility.

- **Efficiency:** Virtual consultations and automated assistance optimise the use of healthcare professionals' time and reduce waiting times for patients.
- **Reduced costs:** Telemedicine can reduce the costs associated with patient travel and medical infrastructure.

- **Continuous care:** Virtual assistance enables continuous monitoring of patients and proactive management of chronic diseases.

- **Saving lives:** In medical emergencies, telemedicine can provide rapid access to medical care and advice, potentially saving lives.

However, it is important to recognise that telemedicine and virtual assistance cannot completely replace traditional healthcare and face-to-face interaction with healthcare professionals. They are designed to complement and improve access to care, while preserving the importance of the carer-patient relationship. Therefore, responsible use of these technologies and a balanced approach are essential to ensure high quality healthcare and a positive patient experience.

Benefits and challenges of AI in frontline care

Artificial intelligence (AI) brings many benefits to the frontline of healthcare, which includes the healthcare professionals who have the first direct contact with patients. Here are some of the key benefits of using AI in this context:

1. Rapid access to medical information: AI can provide instant medical information to healthcare professionals, enabling them to make informed decisions in real time. AI systems can access large databases and continuously update medical knowledge.

2. AI-assisted diagnosis: AI can help healthcare professionals make more accurate diagnoses by analysing complex medical data, such as medical images, test results and medical history. This can speed up the diagnostic process and improve accuracy.

3. Personalised treatment planning: By analysing patient-specific data, AI can develop personalised treatment plans based on each patient's individual characteristics, improving the efficiency of care.

4. Remote patient monitoring: AI enables continuous remote patient monitoring, which is particularly useful for patients suffering from chronic illnesses or convalescing. AI systems can alert healthcare professionals to significant changes in a patient's condition, enabling rapid intervention.

5. Workflow optimisation: AI can automate certain administrative and repetitive tasks, enabling healthcare professionals to focus more on clinical care and reduce their administrative workload.

However, the use of AI in frontline healthcare also presents some challenges:

1. Integration into existing practices: Integrating AI into existing healthcare systems can be complex and requires close collaboration between healthcare professionals and technology experts.

2. Bias and fairness: AI models can be subject to bias, depending on the data they are trained on. It is essential to ensure that models are fair and do not favour certain groups of patients over others.

3. Confidentiality and data security: The use of AI involves the collection and sharing of large amounts of sensitive medical data. Ensuring the confidentiality and security of this data is crucial to protecting patient privacy.

4. Responsibility and accountability: When important medical decisions are made based on AI recommendations, it is essential to determine responsibility in the event of errors or adverse outcomes.

5. Training and skills: Healthcare professionals must be trained in the use of AI and develop specific skills to take full advantage of these technologies.

In summary, AI offers many exciting opportunities to improve the front line of healthcare by enabling more accurate diagnoses, personalised treatments and ongoing patient monitoring. However, addressing the challenges of integration, fairness and privacy is essential to ensure AI is used responsibly and to the benefit of patients and healthcare professionals. An ethical and thoughtful approach is paramount to maximising the benefits of AI while minimising the potential risks.

Strengthening the doctor-patient relationship

The integration of artificial intelligence (AI) into medical practice can actually strengthen the doctor-patient relationship rather than undermine it. Although AI may seem impersonal, it actually offers many benefits that improve communication and the quality of care between doctors and their patients. Here's how AI can strengthen the doctor-patient relationship:

1. More efficient consultation time: By using AI to sort and analyse medical data before the consultation, doctors can spend more time interacting directly with patients. This enables a deeper connection to be established and patient concerns to be addressed in greater depth.

2. Informed decision-making: AI provides doctors with relevant information and evidence-based recommendations, helping them to make more informed decisions about diagnosis and treatment plans. Patients have more confidence in their doctor's decisions when they are supported by evidence and thorough analysis.

3. Personalised treatments: Thanks to AI, doctors can develop personalised treatment plans based on the unique characteristics of each patient. This shows patients that their individual needs are being taken into account, strengthening the relationship of trust with their doctor.

4. Continuous patient monitoring: AI enables continuous remote monitoring of patients, strengthening the doctor-patient relationship by ensuring proactive management of chronic illnesses and ensuring that patients feel supported throughout their care pathway.

5. Improved communication: The use of virtual assistants or chatbots can enable patients to ask questions and obtain medical information at any time, improving communication and access to personalised care.

6. Patient autonomy: AI can provide patients with medical information and educational resources, enabling them to better understand their condition and actively participate in their own care. This empowers patients and encourages a more collaborative relationship with their doctor.

7. Home monitoring: AI can enable patients to monitor their health at home through connected devices and mobile applications. Doctors can track patients' progress remotely, improving their follow-up and engagement in care.

However, it is essential to note that AI can never completely replace the human doctor-patient relationship. The human aspect, empathy and warm communication remain irreplaceable in healthcare. AI must be used responsibly and ethically to complement and enhance the doctor-patient relationship, not to replace it.

In conclusion, the integration of AI into medical practice can strengthen the doctor-patient relationship by improving communication, providing informed medical information and enabling personalised care. AI offers new opportunities to improve the efficiency of care while placing patients at the heart of the decision-making process, thereby strengthening trust and collaboration between healthcare professionals and their patients.

Training and skills for healthcare professionals

With the increasing integration of artificial intelligence (AI) into healthcare, the training and skills of healthcare professionals are becoming essential to take full advantage of these new technologies. Here are some important aspects related to the training of healthcare professionals in the context of AI:

1. Technical training: Healthcare professionals need technical skills to use AI systems effectively and interpret results correctly. This includes learning how to use AI software, understanding machine learning algorithms, and being able to interact with AI tools to obtain relevant patient information.

2. Ethical training: Ethical training is crucial to ensure that healthcare professionals use AI responsibly and fairly. They need to be aware of the ethical challenges associated with the use of AI in healthcare, such as data privacy, algorithmic bias, liability for error and informed decision-making.

3. Adaptability to change: The integration of AI into healthcare represents a major shift in medical practice. Healthcare professionals must be ready to adapt to new technologies and emerging working methods.

4. Continuous training: Given the rapid evolution of AI and its applications in healthcare, continuous training is essential to keep healthcare professionals' skills up to date. This enables them to keep abreast of the latest technological advances and best practices in the field of AI in healthcare.

5. Interdisciplinary collaboration: AI in healthcare often involves collaboration between healthcare professionals and technology experts. It is important that healthcare professionals develop interdisciplinary collaboration skills to work effectively with AI specialists and create synergy between their areas of expertise.

6. Communication skills: Even with the use of AI, communication remains an essential part of healthcare. Healthcare professionals must be able to communicate effectively with their patients in order to establish a relationship of trust and actively involve them in their care.

7. Developing critical thinking skills: Healthcare professionals must be able to understand the results provided by AI critically, checking their accuracy and taking contextual factors into account to avoid errors in diagnosis or treatment.

The training of healthcare professionals in the field of AI should begin with basic studies in medicine, nursing and other healthcare disciplines. Continuing education programmes and professional development workshops can also be set up for practising healthcare professionals. Healthcare institutions and professional organisations have a crucial role to play in facilitating training and providing educational resources to support healthcare professionals in their transition to the effective and ethical use of AI in their clinical practice.

The future of frontline care thanks to AI

The future of frontline healthcare is undeniably linked to artificial intelligence (AI). Rapid advances in AI offer exciting prospects for improving care, increasing the efficiency of medical practices and strengthening the relationship between healthcare professionals and patients. Here's how AI could transform the future of frontline healthcare:

1. **Early and accurate diagnosis:** AI will continue to play a crucial role in improving the early and accurate diagnosis of diseases. Through advanced analysis of medical data, images and symptoms, AI systems will be able to detect subtle signs of disease even before symptoms become obvious.

2. **Personalised treatment:** AI will make it possible to develop personalised treatment plans for each patient, taking into account their individual characteristics, preferences and genetics. Treatments can be precisely tailored to maximise efficacy and minimise side effects.

3. **Virtual assistance for healthcare professionals:** Virtual assistants and chatbots will continue to support healthcare professionals by answering patients' questions, providing medical information and managing appointments. This will allow doctors and nurses to focus more on clinical care.

4. **Widespread telemedicine:** Telemedicine will become an integral part of healthcare, enabling patients to consult their doctors remotely for consultations, medical follow-up and prescriptions, thereby improving access to care.

5. **Proactive management of chronic diseases:** AI systems will enable healthcare professionals to continuously monitor patients with chronic diseases and quickly detect any signs of deterioration, enabling early and proactive management.

6. **Human-machine collaboration:** AI will work closely with healthcare professionals to provide relevant recommendations and information, enabling doctors, nurses and other professionals to make informed decisions and deliver high-quality care.

7. Preventive screening: AI will be used to perform predictive analyses to identify risk factors in patients and identify those who could benefit from preventive screening for potential diseases.

8. Continuing education and specialisation: AI will open up new opportunities for the continuing education and specialisation of healthcare professionals. They will be able to acquire additional skills to use AI technologies effectively in their clinical practice.

However, it is important to note that despite the many advances in AI, the human dimension will remain crucial in healthcare. Patients need compassion, empathy and a relationship of trust with their healthcare professionals. AI must be used responsibly to complement and improve healthcare, while keeping the patient's well-being at the centre of attention.

In summary, the future of frontline healthcare will be shaped by the integration of AI, enabling more accurate diagnosis and treatment, better management of chronic conditions, and an overall improvement in the efficiency of care. To fully grasp the benefits of AI, it is essential to train and prepare healthcare professionals to use this technology responsibly and ethically, while maintaining the importance of the doctor-patient relationship and the human aspect of healthcare.

AI in palliative care: Technological comfort and human support

Introduction to palliative care and AI

Palliative care is a comprehensive approach to healthcare that aims to improve the quality of life of patients with serious illnesses, focusing on the relief of pain, symptoms and emotional suffering. The introduction of artificial intelligence (AI) into palliative care offers new opportunities to improve the care of patients at the end of life and support their families. Here's how AI could be integrated into palliative care:

1. **Symptom management:** AI can be used to monitor end-of-life patients' symptoms, such as pain, nausea or fatigue, in real time. Wearable sensors and connected devices can collect valuable data, helping healthcare professionals adjust treatments for optimal symptom relief.

2. Prediction of patient needs: By analysing medical data and patient history, AI can anticipate the patient's future palliative care needs. This enables proactive planning of interventions and better patient care.

3. Communication support: AI can provide educational resources and medical information to patients and their families, helping them to better understand the disease and the treatment options available. Chatbots or virtual assistants can also be used to answer questions from patients and their loved ones, providing ongoing support throughout the palliative care process.

4. Emotional support: The RN can provide emotional support to patients and their families by offering psychological help resources, stress management techniques and counselling services tailored to their specific needs.

5. Advanced medical directive planning: AI can help patients develop advance medical directives based on their values and preferences. This ensures that patients receive care in line with their wishes, even when their ability to make decisions is impaired.

6. Optimising the use of resources: AI can help optimise the use of resources by efficiently allocating staff and coordinating palliative care services to meet the growing needs of patients at the end of life.

7. Care monitoring and evaluation: AI can be used to evaluate the effectiveness of palliative care and identify areas for improvement. This enables clinical practice to be continually optimised and the quality of care to be improved.

However, it is important to note that AI can never replace the human dimension of palliative care. The essential role of healthcare professionals, nurses and support staff in providing empathetic communication, active listening and emotional support to patients at the end of life and their families cannot be replaced by technology.

In conclusion, the introduction of AI into palliative care offers significant benefits for improving the care of patients at the end of life. AI can contribute to more effective symptom management, better communication and emotional support for patients and their families. However, it is crucial to maintain the importance of the human relationship and compassion in the delivery of palliative care, using AI in complementary ways to optimise the quality of care and improve the overall experience of patients at the end of life.

Pain and symptom relief

Artificial intelligence (AI) offers promising opportunities for pain and symptom relief in healthcare settings, including palliative care. Here's how AI can help improve pain and symptom relief:

1. Real-time monitoring: AI can enable real-time monitoring of patients' symptoms through the use of wearable sensors and connected medical devices. This data is then analysed to provide valuable information on the evolution of pain and other symptoms, allowing healthcare professionals to quickly adjust the treatment plan according to the patient's needs.

2. Early detection: AI can detect early signs of pain or emerging symptoms that may be overlooked by the patient or missed during traditional medical visits. This enables early and proactive intervention to relieve discomfort before it worsens.

3. Personalised analgesia: Using AI, healthcare professionals can design personalised pain management approaches for each patient, taking into account individual characteristics, medical history, response to previous treatments and other factors influencing pain sensitivity.

4. Treatment optimisation: AI can be used to analyse large clinical and research datasets to identify the most effective treatments for certain conditions or symptoms. This allows evidence-based treatment decisions to be made and patients to be offered the best options available to alleviate their symptoms.

5. Crisis prediction: For certain chronic diseases or conditions, AI can anticipate the occurrence of crises or acute episodes, such as pain crises in patients suffering from certain chronic diseases. This enables healthcare professionals to be better prepared to react quickly and relieve patients' pain as soon as possible.

6. Managing polypharmacy: AI can help manage potentially dangerous drug interactions or optimise drug dosages to minimise unwanted side effects, helping to improve patient comfort while minimising risk.

7. Non-pharmacological intervention: AI can also support the use of non-pharmacological interventions, such as music therapy, virtual reality or cognitive behavioural therapy, to relieve pain and symptoms in some patients.

It is important to emphasise that although AI can offer many benefits for pain and symptom relief, it should never replace the relationship between healthcare professional and patient. Empathetic communication and careful listening remain key to fully understanding the patient's experience and adapting care accordingly.

In summary, artificial intelligence offers opportunities to improve pain and symptom relief through real-time monitoring, early detection, personalisation of treatments, and optimisation of interventions. The judicious use of AI, combined with the expertise and compassion of healthcare professionals, can help to significantly improve patients' quality of life, particularly in the context of palliative care and chronic illness.

Personalised care and communications

Artificial intelligence (AI) is opening up exciting possibilities for personalised care and communication in healthcare. By analysing large datasets, AI can provide valuable information about patients and help them make informed healthcare decisions. Here's how AI can be used to personalise care and communications:

1. Patient profiling: AI can analyse patients' medical histories, test results, lifestyle habits and preferences to create individual profiles. These profiles help healthcare professionals to better understand the specific needs of each patient and tailor treatment plans accordingly.

2. Personalised treatment recommendations: Using AI, healthcare professionals can receive personalised treatment recommendations based on the specific characteristics of each patient. This enables more targeted treatment plans to be devised, increasing the chances of success and reducing undesirable side effects.

3. Tailored communication: AI can be used to tailor communication to individual patient needs. For example, some patients may prefer to receive appointment reminders by SMS, while others prefer phone calls or emails. AI can identify the preferred communication channels for each patient, improving communication efficiency.

4. Remote monitoring: Through the use of connected sensors and wearable devices, AI enables remote monitoring of patients. Healthcare professionals can receive real-time data on patients' health, enabling them to detect changes or potential problems more quickly and provide appropriate assistance in a timely manner.

5. Patient education and empowerment: AI can help provide personalised medical information to patients, educating them about their specific health condition and available treatment options. This enables patients to make informed decisions about their health and become active partners in their care.

6. Targeted prevention: By analysing individual risk factors, AI can help identify patients who are most likely to develop certain diseases. This enables early, targeted intervention to prevent or slow disease progression.

7. Chronic disease management: AI can support chronic disease management by providing personalised reminders to take medication, encouraging adherence to treatment regimes and providing advice on lifestyle changes to improve long-term health.

While AI offers exciting opportunities to personalise care and communication, it is essential to recognise that the human dimension remains irreplaceable in the relationship between healthcare professionals and patients. AI should be used in a complementary way to support and improve care, emphasising a patient-centred approach and ensuring that patients' individual needs and preferences are respected.

In conclusion, AI offers innovative ways to personalise healthcare and communications, providing treatment recommendations tailored to each patient, preferred communication channels, and tailored education. The responsible use of AI in healthcare will improve the effectiveness and efficiency of care while strengthening the relationship between patients and healthcare professionals.

Assistance for carers and healthcare professionals

Artificial intelligence (AI) offers considerable potential to provide valuable assistance to carers and healthcare professionals in their role of caring for patients. Using sophisticated algorithms and data analysis, AI can improve care processes, offer relevant information and make administrative tasks easier. Here's how AI can help:

1. Medical records management: AI can be used to organise and manage patients' medical records efficiently. By automating certain administrative tasks related to documentation, AI allows healthcare professionals to spend more time interacting with patients and providing care.

2. Diagnostic support: AI can help healthcare professionals in the diagnostic process by analysing patients' medical data, proposing hypotheses and providing information on possible treatment options. This can be particularly useful for complex or rare diseases.

3. Predicting treatment outcomes: Using AI, healthcare professionals can make predictions about the likely outcomes of proposed treatments. This helps them choose the best treatment approach for each patient, taking into account their specific health condition and medical history.

4. Clinical decision support: AI can provide recommendations and advice to healthcare professionals when faced with complex clinical decisions. These suggestions can be based on scientific evidence, medical protocols and best practice.

5. Remote patient monitoring: AI enables continuous remote patient monitoring through the use of sensors and connected devices. This enables healthcare professionals to rapidly detect any changes in a patient's state of health and intervene accordingly.

6. Emotional support for carers: AI can provide emotional support to carers by offering psychological help resources, stress management strategies and information on patient management.

7. Continuing education: AI can be used to offer continuing education to healthcare professionals, providing them with e-learning modules tailored to their needs and speciality.

8. Resource optimisation: AI can help optimise the use of resources in healthcare establishments by predicting demand, optimising working hours and facilitating care planning.

However, it is important to note that AI should not replace the role of healthcare professionals and carers, but rather support and complement them. The human relationship and compassion remain essential in healthcare, and AI must be used ethically and responsibly to improve care without compromising the relationship between carers and patients.

In conclusion, AI offers many opportunities to assist carers and healthcare professionals by facilitating administrative tasks, improving care processes, providing relevant information and optimising the use of resources. The responsible integration of AI in healthcare can help to improve the efficiency and quality of care while easing the workload of carers.

Limits of AI in palliative care

While artificial intelligence (AI) offers many opportunities to improve palliative care, it also has some limitations that need to be considered. Here are some of the limitations of AI in this context:

1. Complexity of comprehensive care: Palliative care often involves a comprehensive and holistic approach to patient care, which includes not only the relief of physical symptoms, but also emotional, social and spiritual support. Although AI can help with symptom management, it cannot replace the human and empathetic dimension of the overall support provided by healthcare professionals and carers.

2. Understanding emotional needs: AI can provide information about physical symptoms and disease progression, but it may struggle to understand the emotional and psychological needs of patients at the end of life. Empathetic communication and human connection remain essential to meet the emotional needs of patients and their families.

3. Ethical decision-making: AI can provide evidence-based treatment recommendations, but there may be complex situations where ethical decisions cannot be made on the basis of data alone. Ethical decision-making in palliative care requires careful consideration, taking into account the patient's values and preferences, which is beyond the scope of AI.

4. Confidentiality and data protection: The use of AI in palliative care involves the collection and processing of sensitive patient health data. Ensuring the confidentiality and protection of this data is essential to maintain trust between patients, carers and healthcare professionals.

5. Cost and accessibility: Some AI technologies can be expensive to implement and maintain, which may limit their accessibility for some less developed healthcare settings or regions. It is essential to ensure that the adoption of AI in palliative care is equitable and accessible to all patients, regardless of where they live or their economic circumstances.

6. Technological dependency: While AI offers significant benefits, over-reliance on technology can lead to risks, including the dehumanisation of care, reduced human decision-making and loss of connection between patients and carers.

7. Continuous learning: AI relies on learning from past data. It is therefore essential to ensure that AI models are regularly updated and reflect current medical advances and best practice.

In conclusion, while AI offers exciting opportunities to improve palliative care, it also has limitations that are important to consider. The key lies in responsibly integrating AI into palliative care, emphasising the human dimension and ensuring that care decisions take into account both medical data and the emotional and ethical needs of patients and their families.

Integrative approach: Combining AI with human support

The integrative approach involves combining artificial intelligence (AI) with human support to deliver comprehensive, high-quality healthcare. Rather than seeking to completely replace healthcare professionals with AI, this approach aims to harness the respective strengths of AI and human expertise to improve patient care and experience. Here's how this approach can be implemented in different facets of healthcare:

1. AI-assisted diagnosis with human confirmation: AI can be used to rapidly analyse huge amounts of medical data and propose diagnostic hypotheses. Healthcare professionals can then examine these diagnostic suggestions, taking into account their own expertise and all the patient's information to confirm or adjust the diagnosis.

2. Personalised treatment plans: AI can provide recommendations based on medical protocols and evidence for the management of a specific disease. Healthcare professionals can then personalise these recommendations by taking into account the patient's preferences, general health, values and goals.

3. Continuous patient monitoring: AI can be used to monitor patients' vital signs and symptoms remotely in real time. If any worrying changes are detected, AI can alert healthcare professionals for immediate, personalised intervention.

4. Emotional support and empathic communication: Although AI can be useful for providing information and reminders, there is no substitute for the emotional support and empathic communication provided by healthcare professionals and carers. They can create bonds with patients, understand their emotions and respond to their psychological needs.

5. Shared decision-making: AI can help provide objective information about treatment options and their likely outcomes. However, the final decision making should always be shared between the patient and the healthcare professional, taking into account the patient's values and preferences.

6. Continuing education for healthcare professionals: AI can be used as a continuing education tool for healthcare professionals, providing them with updates on the latest medical advances and new treatment approaches.

7. Privacy and ethics: The integrative approach must take account of ethical issues and the protection of patient privacy, ensuring that medical data is used responsibly and securely.

By integrating AI ethically and responsibly into healthcare, we can improve the efficiency and accuracy of care while maintaining a strong human connection between healthcare professionals, patients and their families. This integrative approach makes the most of AI technologies while valuing the expertise and compassion of carers, for more comprehensive, personalised and patient-centred healthcare.

Outlook for the future : The evolution of palliative care with AI

The prospects for the future of palliative care with artificial intelligence (AI) are promising and are generating a great deal of interest in the healthcare field. AI has the potential to significantly transform the delivery of palliative care by improving the efficiency, quality and accessibility of services offered to patients at the end of life. Here are some key perspectives for the evolution of palliative care with AI:

1. Improved accuracy of diagnosis and prediction: By analysing large sets of medical data, AI can help improve the accuracy of diagnosis of serious diseases and end-of-life conditions. It can also more accurately predict disease progression and future patient needs, enabling more effective care planning.

2. Personalised care: AI can be used to provide more personalised palliative care by taking into account the unique characteristics of each patient. Treatment plans can be tailored according to each individual's preferences, values and goals, improving quality of life at the end of life.

3. Continuous patient monitoring: AI enables continuous monitoring of patients at the end of life, even remotely, through the use of sensors and connected devices. This enables healthcare professionals to rapidly detect any changes in the patient's state of health and provide appropriate intervention in a timely manner.

4. Emotional and psychological support: AI can be used to provide emotional support to patients and their families at the end of life. Empathetic chatbots and virtual support programmes can help meet patients' emotional needs and provide psychological support resources.

5. Patient and family education: AI can be used to provide educational information to patients and their families about palliative care, treatment options, ethical decisions and symptom management. This allows patients to be more involved in their care and facilitates shared decision-making.

6. Integrating palliative care into healthcare systems: AI can help to further integrate palliative care into healthcare systems by facilitating the sharing of information between different care providers and healthcare institutions. This helps to ensure smoother continuity of care for patients at the end of life.

7. Research and development of new treatments: AI can accelerate medical research in palliative care by rapidly analysing large amounts of data and identifying potential new therapeutic targets. This could lead to major advances in the treatment of severe symptoms and illnesses at the end of life.

It is important to stress that, despite the positive outlook, AI must never replace the human dimension in palliative care. The presence and emotional support of healthcare professionals and carers remain essential in providing a comprehensive and empathetic approach to end-of-life care.

In conclusion, AI offers many opportunities to improve palliative care, by increasing diagnostic accuracy, personalising treatments, offering emotional support and facilitating access to care. The responsible integration of AI into palliative care can help improve the quality of life of patients at the end of life and support their families throughout this difficult period. However, it is essential to ensure that AI is used in an ethical and patient-centred way, always keeping compassion and empathy at the heart of palliative care.

The future of healthcare:
An integrated vision of AI and humanity

Introduction to the future of healthcare

The future of healthcare promises to be marked by technological advances and innovations that will profoundly transform the way healthcare services are delivered. Several key factors will help shape this exciting future:

1. Artificial Intelligence (AI) and Big Data: AI and Big Data analysis will play a key role in tomorrow's healthcare. AI can help improve diagnosis, clinical decision-making, medical records management, disease prediction, and facilitate medical research. Massive data will also enable a better understanding of health trends, epidemics and disease patterns.

2. Telemedicine and digital health: Telemedicine will continue to develop, offering patients access to healthcare at a distance, overcoming geographical barriers and reducing waiting times. Health applications, wearable devices and connected sensors will play an increasing role in monitoring and managing people's health.

3. Personalised care: Advances in genomics, precision medicine and AI will enable more personalised healthcare tailored to the specific characteristics of each patient. Treatments will be tailored to the genetic profile and unique needs of each individual.

4. Robotics and automation: Medical robotics will continue to develop, supporting healthcare professionals in surgical tasks, rehabilitation, patient care and hospital logistics. Automation will help to increase process efficiency, reduce errors and free up time for quality care.

5. Regenerative medicine: Research into regenerative medicine will progress, making it possible to regenerate damaged tissues and organs. This will open up possibilities for treating certain chronic diseases and serious injuries.

6. Ethics and security: As technology advances, the issue of ethics and health data protection will become increasingly crucial. Strict ethical standards will need to be put in place to guarantee the confidentiality and security of patient information.

7. Interdisciplinary collaboration: The future of healthcare will require greater collaboration between healthcare professionals, researchers, engineers and technology experts. Together, they will be able to develop innovative solutions to healthcare challenges.

8. Ongoing training: Healthcare professionals will need regular training in new technologies and emerging practices in order to remain up to date in their field and offer quality care.

In short, the future of healthcare will be characterised by a more personalised, technological and patient-centred approach. Technological advances such as AI, telemedicine and regenerative medicine will offer opportunities for more efficient, accessible and prevention-focused healthcare. However, it will be essential to ensure that these advances are used responsibly, ethically and fairly to maximise the benefits for society as a whole.

AI as a complement to carers

Artificial intelligence (AI) is set to become a valuable adjunct to healthcare workers. Rather than completely replacing healthcare professionals, AI can be strategically integrated to improve their efficiency, decision-making and care delivery. Here's how AI can act as an essential complement to caregivers:

1. AI-assisted data analysis and diagnosis: AI can rapidly process huge amounts of medical data, including medical images, electronic records and test results. This capability enables healthcare professionals to access more complete information and to be assisted in the diagnostic process. AI can provide evidence-based treatment recommendations, enabling doctors to make more informed decisions.

2. Continuous patient monitoring: AI can be used to monitor patients' vital signs and health data remotely in real time. Carers can be alerted to any worrying changes, enabling them to intervene quickly and avoid complications.

3. Medical records management: AI can automate the management of medical records, recording relevant information, monitoring treatments and facilitating coordination between different care providers. This allows carers to focus more on the direct delivery of care.

4. Assistance with repetitive tasks: AI can be used to automate repetitive and administrative tasks, such as scheduling appointments, billing and managing medication stocks. This allows carers to save time and focus on more complex and engaging tasks.

5. Continuing education and training: AI can be used as a continuing education tool for carers, providing updates on the latest medical advances, treatment protocols and best practice. This enables healthcare professionals to keep abreast of the latest innovations and continually improve their skills.

6. Emotional support for patients and carers: AI can be used to provide emotional support to patients and carers, offering virtual support programmes, empathetic chatbots and stress management resources. This can help relieve the emotional burden on carers and improve patient wellbeing.

7. Medical research: AI can accelerate medical research by analysing large datasets and identifying new avenues of research. This can lead to important medical discoveries and new treatments for patients.

By integrating AI ethically and responsibly, carers can harness its benefits to improve the quality of care, increase efficiency and enhance the overall patient experience. However, it is important to stress that AI cannot completely replace the human expertise and compassion of carers. The relationship of trust between patients and carers remains essential to providing quality, patient-centred care. AI should be used in a complementary way, helping carers to do their jobs better rather than replacing them, to ensure an optimal balance between technology and humanity in healthcare.

AI for resource and cost management

Artificial intelligence (AI) offers numerous opportunities to improve the management of resources and costs in the healthcare sector. Here are a few areas where AI can play a key role in this management:

1. Workforce and resource planning: AI can be used to analyse attendance data and seasonal trends in healthcare facilities, enabling more accurate workforce and resource planning. This helps to avoid understaffing or overstaffing, while maintaining optimum quality of care.

2. Schedule optimisation: AI can optimise staff schedules by taking into account the specific skills of healthcare professionals, their availability and the needs of patients. This reduces downtime and improves operational efficiency.

3. Hospital bed management: AI can help predict hospital bed occupancy rates based on expected admissions, expected lengths of stay and patient care needs. This leads to better bed management and reduced waiting times.

4. Process optimisation: AI can analyse hospital processes and identify inefficiencies or bottlenecks. By optimising workflows and automating certain tasks, healthcare establishments can reduce costs and improve the quality of care.

5. Predicting treatment costs: By analysing patient medical data and treatment results, AI can help predict future treatment costs for specific conditions. This enables healthcare establishments and insurers to better anticipate expenditure and better manage budgets.

6. Fraud and billing error detection: AI can be used to detect fraud and billing errors in healthcare systems by analysing billing data and identifying suspicious patterns.

7. Inventory and supply management: AI can predict the need for drugs and medical supplies based on demand trends and current stock levels. This enables more efficient stock management and avoids shortages or surpluses.

8. Tracking population health costs: AI can track population health costs on large scales, identifying factors that influence health costs and recommending chronic disease management strategies.

By using AI for resource and cost management, healthcare organisations can improve operational efficiency, reduce unnecessary costs and deliver better quality care. However, it is important to stress that the introduction of AI in resource management must be done in an ethical and responsible manner, taking into account the implications on patient privacy and ensuring the security and confidentiality of healthcare data. AI should be used as a complementary tool to support healthcare professionals in their decisions and actions, and not as a complete replacement for their expertise and clinical judgement.

Training and preparation for tomorrow's healthcare

Training and preparing healthcare professionals for tomorrow's healthcare is essential if they are to adapt to technological advances and new approaches to medicine. Here are a few key points concerning training and preparation for tomorrow's healthcare:

1. Integration of technology and AI skills: Healthcare training programmes should include modules on technology skills, the use of AI in healthcare and the analysis of medical data. Future healthcare professionals should be trained to use emerging technologies to improve care and clinical decision-making.

2. Continuing education and retraining: Continuing education is crucial to enable healthcare professionals to keep up to date with the latest medical and technological advances. Retraining opportunities should be offered on a regular basis to develop new skills and deepen knowledge.

3. Interdisciplinary training: Tomorrow's healthcare will involve close collaboration between different disciplines, including healthcare professionals, engineers, researchers and technology experts. Interdisciplinary training will enable future healthcare professionals to better understand different perspectives and to work effectively as part of a team.

4. Learning by doing: Learning by doing, through placements and clinical rotations, is crucial to enable medical students and other health professionals to develop practical skills and become familiar with new medical technologies.

5. Ethics and security training: Future healthcare professionals should be trained in the ethics of using AI and technology in healthcare. They should also be made aware of data security and patient confidentiality issues.

6. Developing communication and empathy skills: As technology continues to play an increasing role in healthcare, it is essential that healthcare professionals develop communication and empathy skills to maintain a trusting relationship with patients.

7. Encouraging innovation and curiosity: Training programmes should encourage innovation and curiosity in future healthcare professionals. This will foster a spirit of exploration and openness to new ideas and approaches.

8. Developing digital health leaders: It will be important to develop digital health leaders who can lead and oversee the implementation of new technologies and digital solutions in healthcare institutions.

By preparing healthcare professionals for tomorrow's healthcare, we can ensure that they are ready to meet the challenges of the future and take advantage of the opportunities offered by technological advances. Continuing education, the integration of technology skills and a focus on ethics and communication will be key to creating a skilled healthcare workforce capable of delivering high quality, patient-centred care in an ever-changing healthcare environment.

Data security and confidentiality in the future of healthcare

Data security and privacy will play a crucial role in the future of healthcare as technological advances, including artificial intelligence (AI) and the increased use of medical data, continue to reshape the sector. Here are some key points to bear in mind about data security and privacy in the future of healthcare:

1. Protection of patient data : Patients' medical data contains sensitive information about their health and privacy. It is essential that robust security measures are put in place to protect this data from unauthorised access or theft. This includes the use of encryption, strong authentication and firewalls to prevent data breaches.

2. Cybersecurity risk management: As the healthcare sector becomes increasingly digitised, cybersecurity risks also increase. Healthcare organisations will need to invest in sophisticated IT security systems to protect against cyber attacks, ransomware and other potential threats.

3. Informed consent and data control: Patients should have control over their medical data and be informed of how that data will be used. Informed consent must be obtained for any use or sharing of medical data, and patients should be able to withdraw their consent at any time.

4. Integrating data protection by design: When developing new healthcare technologies and applications, data protection should be integrated by design (Privacy by Design). This means that confidentiality and security considerations must be taken into account right from the start of the development process.

5. Healthcare staff training: Healthcare professionals will need to be trained on data security practices and how to protect patient information. Ongoing training will be required to make staff aware of new threats and best practices in data security.

6. Compliance with data protection regulations: Healthcare facilities will need to comply with data protection regulations, such as the General Data Protection Regulation (GDPR) in Europe and the Health Insurance Portability and Accountability Act (HIPAA) in the US. These regulations set strict standards for the collection, storage and use of medical data.

7. Liability in the event of a data breach: In the event of a data breach, it is essential to establish accountability and to inform affected patients promptly. Healthcare organisations will need to have incident response plans in place to effectively manage data breaches and minimise the impact on patients.

By putting robust security and privacy measures in place, healthcare will be able to take full advantage of the benefits of AI and new technologies while protecting patients' rights and privacy. Patient trust in the healthcare system is essential to ensure successful uptake and collaboration, and this can only be achieved through responsible and ethical management of health data.

Reflecting on the importance of humanity in healthcare

The importance of humanity in healthcare cannot be underestimated. Despite technological advances and the increasing integration of artificial intelligence into healthcare, the human element remains essential to providing high-quality, patient-centred care. Here are some thoughts on the importance of humanity in healthcare:

1. The carer-patient relationship : The relationship between carer and patient is fundamental to establishing trust, empathy and emotional support. Human contact, attentive listening and compassion play an essential role in patients' recovery and well-being.

2. Understanding individual needs: Healthcare professionals can provide personalised care by assessing the unique needs of each patient. They can take into account the social, emotional and environmental factors that influence an individual's health, which is not always possible for AI.

3. Ethical decision-making: Healthcare often involves complex, sometimes ethical, decisions where AI may not be able to fully understand the nuances and personal values of patients. Healthcare professionals contribute their ethical judgement and expertise to make responsible and informed decisions.

4. Managing emotions : The healthcare experience can be emotionally challenging for patients and their families. Healthcare professionals play a crucial role in providing emotional support, responding to concerns and empathising with patients' emotions.

5. Adaptability and flexibility: Human carers are able to adapt to unexpected situations, react to subtle changes in a patient's condition and be creative in responding to changing needs. This adaptability is a unique quality that AI may struggle to replicate.

6. Complex communication: Communication between patients and carers often involves complex and nuanced exchanges. Healthcare professionals are trained to interpret patients' verbal and non-verbal cues, which can be difficult for AI that relies primarily on textual or numerical data.

7. Cultural sensitivity: Healthcare must be adapted to patients' cultural values and beliefs. Healthcare professionals can develop cultural sensitivity to provide respectful and appropriate care to diverse populations, which is crucial in an increasingly diverse world.
Although AI and medical technologies can bring significant improvements to healthcare, they cannot replace the human aspect. The presence of human carers is irreplaceable in providing emotional support, making complex decisions, responding to individual needs and developing a relationship of trust with patients.

In the future of healthcare, it is essential to maintain a balance between technological advances and the humanity of care. Technology should be used as a complementary tool to support healthcare professionals in their work, rather than replacing them. This ensures that care remains patient-centred, respectful and holistic, providing a more satisfying overall healthcare experience for patients and carers.

Conclusion: Forging an integrated future for AI and humanity in healthcare

The convergence of artificial intelligence (AI) and humanity in healthcare is opening up an exciting and promising future. As technologies continue to develop and transform the medical landscape, it is essential to forge an integrated future where AI and humanity work in synergy to deliver optimal, patient-centric healthcare. Here are some key points for shaping this integrated future:

1. Collaboration between AI and human carers: Rather than seeing AI as a threat to human carers, it is essential to promote a culture of collaboration and partnership between the two. AI can complement the skills and expertise of healthcare professionals by providing information and decision support tools, enabling them to deliver more accurate and personalised care.

2. Focus on the carer-patient relationship: Although AI can automate certain tasks, the human relationship remains at the heart of healthcare. Healthcare professionals must continue to place great importance on active listening, empathy and compassion in order to establish a relationship of trust with patients. AI can free up time for carers so that they can focus more on the relational aspect of care.

3. Ethical and responsible integration of AI: As AI continues to advance, it is crucial that it is integrated ethically and responsibly into healthcare. This includes protecting data privacy, making algorithms transparent, avoiding bias and ensuring patient safety. Regulations and ethical standards must be put in place to guide the use of AI in healthcare.

4. Training and skills development: Healthcare professionals need to be trained in new AI technologies and skills, while maintaining a solid foundation of medical knowledge and human skills. Training programmes should favour an interdisciplinary approach and encourage continuous learning to adapt to constant developments in the field.

5. Investment in research and innovation: To shape an integrated future of AI and humanity in healthcare, continued investment in research and innovation is essential. Technological advances must be supported by rigorous research to evaluate their effectiveness and impact on patient outcomes.

6. Patient-centricity: In all developments and applications of AI in healthcare, the patient must remain the focus. Technologies and innovations must be designed to meet patients' needs, improve their quality of life and help them make informed decisions about their health.

By combining the unique capabilities of AI with the human qualities of caregivers, we can create a powerful and complementary healthcare ecosystem. AI can improve efficiency, accuracy and access to care, while humanity brings the compassion, ethical decision-making and empathy essential to delivering high-quality care.

In conclusion, the integrated future of AI and humanity in healthcare relies on a harmonious collaboration between emerging technologies and human caregivers. By capitalising on the strengths of each field, we can positively transform the healthcare landscape, delivering more efficient and patient-centred care, while ensuring the security and confidentiality of medical data. By maintaining an ethical approach, valuing the carer-patient relationship and continuing to promote innovation, we will shape an integrated and sustainable future for healthcare.

Conclusion

Summary of the book's main arguments.

The book explores the emerging role of artificial intelligence (AI) in healthcare and focuses on the central question: "Can artificial intelligence ever replace the carer?" Here is a summary of the main arguments developed throughout the book:

1. Benefits of AI in healthcare: The book highlights the many benefits of AI in healthcare, including increased accuracy in diagnosis, more informed clinical decision-making, efficient management of medical data and improved patient monitoring.

2. The importance of emotional intelligence and human skills: The book emphasises the crucial importance of emotional intelligence and human skills in the carer-patient relationship. It highlights the fact that empathy, warm communication and the ability to provide emotional support remain essential to providing comprehensive, patient-centred care.

3. Harmonious cohabitation between AI and the human caregiver: Rather than completely replacing the human caregiver, AI can be used as a complementary tool to enhance the caregiver's capabilities and performance. The book stresses the importance of a harmonious cohabitation between AI and human skills to provide optimal healthcare.

4. AI as a "colleague" to the carer: The book explores the prospect of AI acting as a 'colleague' to the carer rather than a replacement. AI can free up time and resources for carers, allowing them to focus on more complex and relational aspects of care.

5. Ethical challenges and liability: The book addresses the ethical dilemmas associated with the use of AI in healthcare, such as data confidentiality, transparency in AI decision-making and liability in the event of errors or misinterpretations.

6. Successful integration of AI: The book proposes strategies for successful integration of AI into existing care practices, including a focus on training healthcare professionals, collaboration between AI and human caregivers, and validation and transparency of AI models.

7. Impact on healthcare training and the evolution of professions: The book explores the potential impact of AI on healthcare training, highlighting the need for AI and technology-driven training, as well as the development of new complementary skills.

In summary, the book presents an in-depth analysis of the implications of artificial intelligence in healthcare. It highlights the benefits of AI while emphasising the continued importance of emotional intelligence and human skills in the delivery of quality healthcare. It proposes approaches for the successful integration of AI into healthcare practices, while addressing the ethical issues and challenges associated with this technological evolution. Finally, it considers the evolution of the medical professions and the importance of continuing education to enable healthcare professionals to adapt to these changes.

Answer to the initial question: Will AI one day replace the carer?

The answer to the initial question of whether artificial intelligence (AI) will one day replace the carer is complex and nuanced. To date, AI has shown promising potential to improve healthcare, but it is unlikely to completely replace the role of the human carer.

1. Complementary role of AI: AI can be used as a complementary tool to enhance the capabilities of human caregivers. It can help perform repetitive tasks, analyse huge amounts of data, provide evidence-based recommendations and facilitate clinical decision-making. This will allow caregivers to focus more on patient interaction, the emotional aspect of care and complex decisions requiring human intuition.

2. Importance of emotional intelligence: Emotional intelligence and human skills are essential elements of the caregiver-patient relationship. Human carers are capable of empathy, compassion and a deep understanding of patients' emotional needs. These qualities cannot be replicated by AI, and therein lies their unique value in delivering high-quality healthcare.

3. Complexity of clinical decision-making: Clinical decision-making in complex and unpredictable situations requires human expertise, based on clinical experience, intuition and the ability to weigh up ethical considerations. AI can provide information and recommendations, but the overall assessment of the medical context and the final decision-making rests with the human caregiver.

4. Accountability and trust: Accountability and trust are crucial factors in healthcare. Patients need to be able to trust their carer to make informed decisions and support them through their care journey. AI raises questions about accountability in the event of errors or misinterpretations, reinforcing the importance of human presence to take responsibility for clinical decisions.

5. Changing roles: The integration of AI into healthcare is likely to change the traditional roles of healthcare professionals. Carers may focus more on the relational, emotional and educational aspects of care, while AI supports certain technical and administrative tasks.

In conclusion, although artificial intelligence is playing an increasingly important role in healthcare, it will not completely replace the human carer. The harmonious cohabitation of AI and human skills is the key to delivering superior healthcare, combining the power of technology with the essence of compassion and humanity in healthcare. The carer-patient relationship remains deeply rooted in emotional intelligence, understanding and support, ensuring that AI becomes a valuable complement to, but never a substitute for, the essential role of the human carer.

Final message on the importance of responsible innovation and humanity in healthcare.

The final message of this book highlights the crucial importance of responsible innovation and humanity in healthcare. As artificial intelligence (AI) and advanced technologies open up exciting new perspectives in healthcare, it is essential to keep ethical principles in mind and preserve the very essence of humanity in medical practice.

1. Ethical responsibility: When integrating AI into healthcare, it is essential to focus on ethical responsibility. Decisions about patients should never be entirely delegated to AI, but rather guided by the ethical values and medical knowledge of healthcare professionals. We must continually assess the impact of AI on patients, data confidentiality and equity in access to care.

2. Personalised care: While AI can help provide evidence-based recommendations and treatments, it is essential to consider each patient as a unique individual. Humanity in healthcare is about taking into account each patient's preferences, values and personal circumstances to develop personalised treatment plans.

3. Human and technological collaboration: Responsible innovation in healthcare means seeking harmonious collaboration between human carers and advanced technologies. AI can relieve repetitive and administrative tasks, allowing carers to spend more time interacting with patients, empathising and communicating.

4. Strengthening the carer-patient relationship: AI should not be a barrier in the carer-patient relationship, but rather a catalyst to strengthen that relationship. Technology should be used to improve care and understanding between healthcare professionals and patients, creating an environment of trust and support.

5. Informed decision-making: Healthcare professionals need to be informed about the capabilities and limitations of AI. Responsible innovation requires ongoing education and appropriate training for caregivers to help them interpret AI results, understand its implications and make informed decisions.

6. Never lose sight of humanity: While technological advances are advancing rapidly, it is crucial never to lose sight of the humanity at the heart of healthcare. Patients need compassion, emotional support and holistic care, and these can only be provided by human carers with emotional intelligence and interpersonal skills.

In conclusion, responsible innovation and humanity are two essential pillars for the future of healthcare. Artificial intelligence and advanced technologies can certainly improve care, but they must be used ethically, responsibly and in a way that complements human skills. We must continue to put patients at the centre of medical practice, recognising the fundamental importance of the carer-patient relationship and preserving the compassion and humanity that make healthcare such a unique and essential profession. By embracing responsible innovation and preserving humanity, we can shape a future where technology improves care while strengthening the precious bond between carers and their patients.